# Yoga for Pelvic Floor and Postpartum Health

# YOGA for PELVIC FLOOR and POSTPARTUM HEALTH

An Iyengar Yoga Approach to
Pelvic Healing and Integrative Wellness
through Anatomy and Practice

**Meagen Satinsky, MPT**
and **Rebecca Weisman, CIYT**

North Atlantic Books
Huichin, unceded Ohlone land
Berkeley, California

Published by
North Atlantic Books
Huichin, unceded Ohlone land
Berkeley, California

Photos by Arik Cardenas
Cover design by Mimi Bark
Book design by Happenstance Type-O-Rama

Printed in the United States of America

*Yoga for Pelvic Floor and Postpartum Health: An Iyengar Yoga Approach to Pelvic Healing and Integrative Wellness through Anatomy and Practice* is sponsored and published by North Atlantic Books, an educational nonprofit based in the unceded Ohlone land Huichin (Berkeley, CA) that collaborates with partners to develop cross-cultural perspectives; nurture holistic views of art, science, the humanities, and healing; and seed personal and global transformation by publishing work on the relationship of body, spirit, and nature.

North Atlantic Books's publications are distributed to the US trade and internationally by Penguin Random House Publisher Services. For further information, visit our website at www.northatlantic books.com.

Library of Congress Cataloging-in-Publication Data

Names: Satinsky, Meagen, 1976- author. | Weisman, Rebecca, 1982- author.
Title: Yoga for pelvic floor and postpartum health : an Iyengar Yoga
    approach to pelvic healing and integrative wellness through anatomy and
    practice / Meagen Satinsky, MPT and Rebecca Weisman, CIYT.
Description: Berkeley, California : North Atlantic Books, [2024] | Includes
    bibliographical references and index. | Summary: "The first
    comprehensive anatomy and yoga practice manual for postpartum pelvic
    healing-a gender-inclusive guide to poses, practices, and exercises for
    pelvic-floor, pain, dysfunction, and recovery"-- Provided by publisher.
Identifiers: LCCN 2023046165 (print) | LCCN 2023046166 (ebook) | ISBN
    9781623179823 (paperback) | ISBN 9781623179830 (epub)
Subjects: LCSH: Postnatal care. | Hatha yoga. | Pelvic floor. | Postnatal
    exercise.
Classification: LCC RG801 .S28 2024  (print) | LCC RG801  (ebook) | DDC
    618.6--dc23/eng/20240301
LC record available at https://lccn.loc.gov/2023046165
LC ebook record available at https://lccn.loc.gov/2023046166

1 2 3 4 5 6 7 8 9 Versa 28 27 26 25 24

North Atlantic Books is committed to the protection of our environment. We print on recycled paper whenever possible and partner with printers who strive to use environmentally responsible practices.

*We joyfully dedicate this book to students past and present whose willingness to share their personal experiences have deeply informed our understanding and the teachings presented in this text.*

# Contents

## Special Topics

# Foreword

Yoga is for one and all. It is a boon at any age or stage of a person's life. For many women, there is an additional facet of motherhood that brings with it both great challenges and joys. This book, *Yoga for Pelvic Floor and Postpartum Health,* is an excellent endeavor to address the needs of new mothers with regard to regaining their energy and strength.

The instructions are lucid and beautifully supported with illustrative photographs. This makes it a very useful resource for practitioners and beginners alike. I am sure this will be a great help to those who do not have easy access to an Iyengar Yoga teacher. There is no substitute for the personal guidance of an experienced teacher, and the practitioner stands to gain immensely from such direct study.

Ultimately, one has to realize that there are many routes to yoga. An approach from the lens of postpartum requirements is but one way. One can liken the pelvic floor approach to being like one petal of the eight limbed Ashtanga Yoga, a starting point. Guruji B. K. S. Iyengar's legacy has been a shining light for practitioners to progress from wherever they may be in their yoga journey. I sincerely wish for this to be a stepping stone to a greater exploration of the holistic science, art, and philosophy of yoga. I am sure this work will help many new parents.

*Abhijata Iyengar*

# Preface

## Personal Notes from the Authors

My relationship with my own pelvis began in my early twenties as I struggled with healing from chronic pelvic pain and urinary disorders. Years later, as I was preparing to give birth to my first child and during the months that followed his birth, I again became interested in the pelvis and pelvic floor muscles and the changes I was experiencing in my body. By that time I was an avid practitioner and yoga teacher, but I was surprised at how much my body changed during this time. Despite feeling confident and knowledgeable, I was surprised by how much of what I was going through felt outside my scope of experience and difficult to grasp or connect to. What a mysterious process pregnancy and childbirth are!

The postpartum time was especially difficult, and healing was slow and compounded by the many demands of becoming a new parent and caring for a newborn. I was reminded of my old pains and suffering. I often felt frustrated and astonished: If someone like me who has so many resources, tools, and knowledge could feel so unprepared, how must others be feeling? This empowered me to learn more about what was happening to my body, and to help others connect to their own pelvis and to heal from pain.

The birth of my second child brought a whole new set of experiences and challenges, and again I was thrown back into eagerly learning about these new pains and symptoms. This made me appreciate the scope of pregnancy, postpartum healing, and the variety of different challenges that people can experience. No two people and no two pregnancies fit into the same box, making an individualized approach essential.

All of this learning has been poured into the courses that Meagen Satinsky and I teach on Postpartum and Pelvic Floor Yoga. Our courses have attracted not only postpartum people, but those who struggle with pelvic floor symptoms and pain, or have experienced changes in their pelvic floor due to menopause and aging. We have learned so much from our students, many of whom are teachers themselves, and continue to grow this vast and much-needed body of knowledge. Like so many, I am drawn to yoga as a deep inquiry into the movements, fluctuations, pains, and joyous mysteries of the body. We offer this book as just one tool to help you begin or deepen your own pelvic floor journey.

*Rebecca Weisman*

The topic of pelvic health was underexplored in my initial physical therapy training and included exactly one lecture. I was surprised that there was only one lecture for an area of the body that is so basic to the human experience and so incredibly important to our continued evolution. In addition, most of what I learned focused solely on pelvic strengthening and Kegels, leaving much to be understood and explored. My own experience included a frightening back injury, which led to my exploration of yoga with an aim at fixing my physical issues. I began to understand that there is more to the body than only the physical realm.

Through my exploration of yoga I began to tap into that knowledge and also to apply these ideas at work with my clients. I immediately noticed a significant shift in the outcomes and results of this work. Through consistent effort and education, my back issues improved, but I was still experiencing one or two debilitating episodes that threw my life into ethical and physical chaos; can I still work, why can't I move properly, how can I fix what's wrong with me, and can I help others even though I myself am suffering?

It was around this time that I took my first pelvic health course. And while it was overwhelming to shift my perspective and learn new vocabulary, I understood that what I was experiencing was going to be greatly improved through the connectivity and applicability of pelvic health science. This was what began my pelvic health journey in earnest. Since then, I have been close to many friends and family members experiencing pregnancy and the effects of pregnancy, birth, and postpartum recovery on their physical, mental, and emotional health. Knowing that pregnancy was something I was not going to choose, I wanted to continue to understand, decipher, and deliver pelvic health science to help serve the many people who could benefit from it.

The opportunity to collaborate with Rebecca on this topic, to help people navigate the challenges and processes of pregnancy, childbirth, and the postpartum period armed with a better canon of knowledge, to share more resources and contribute to a better understanding and management of what is happening in their bodies and with their emotional and mental well-being, is a gift that keeps on giving.

*Meagen Satinsky*

# Acknowledgments

We are honored and excited to share this important resource with you, and with prayers for divine blessings we embark on an exploration of an Iyengar Yoga approach to pelvic floor and postpartum health. We are deeply indebted to B. K. S. Iyengar, whose light continues to shine on, as well as the entire Iyengar family. We honor Geeta Iyengar and Abhijata Iyengar, who continue to be an unparalleled source of knowledge, inspiration, and healing. Abhijata Iyengar's experience as not only the torchbearer of the Iyengar lineage but also a compassionate mother of two children is an inspiration to any yogi who finds themselves seeking their yoga practice as a place of refuge and healing.

We are grateful for the work and guidance of many teachers and helpers in this project. We would also like to thank Rita Keller and Kerstin Khattab, whose book *Iyengar Yoga for Motherhood* has been a constant resource and companion. We also acknowledge the work of Lois Steinberg, whose book *Geeta S. Iyengar's Guide to a Woman's Yoga Practice* offers a valuable treasure trove of information. We would like to thank Patricia Walden, whose teaching, guidance, and compassion is a beacon of light. Thank you to Anthony Grudin for his initial encouragement and Emily Copeland, Alison Aiken, Karen Bumpus, Stephanie Graaf, and Shannon Rodner for editorial support. Thank you to Leslie Freyberg for her help with Sanskrit terms. Finally, we would like to thank our production team: Hannah Wall, Steph Salmon, our three joyful models Hope Elliott, Val Rios, and Sonia Dovedy, and our photographer, Arik Cardenas. Their generous help with this project was exceptional and indispensable.

# Introduction

## Who Is This For?

The sequences in this course are designed to be practiced by people who are newly or not so newly postpartum, those with pelvic floor pain, tightness, or instability, those experiencing pelvic floor symptoms like incontinence or organ prolapse, people going through perimenopause, menopause, or who are postmenopausal, or those who simply want to learn more about the wonders of their own pelvic floor. The content of this book has developed over many years through intensive courses that we have taught on the subject. We often hear the question, "Can I take the class if I'm not postpartum?" The answer is always yes! The pelvic floor is an important part of the body whether or not you've experienced pregnancy and childbirth. It has a close relationship to many other systems and structures in the body and plays a big role in how we breath and walk, and in our posture. It can play a part in spinal and hip health, digestion, sexual and reproductive systems, and the health of the organs.

Our approach to healing the pelvic floor is inclusive, and while students may be coming to the learning from a variety of backgrounds, our approach to healing follows an overall arc that can be helpful to anyone while giving room for variations, flexibility in approach, and modifications. We have worked with students with a wide range of symptoms, life experiences, and abilities, and the material in this book will provide something for everyone. We give in-depth anatomical descriptions coupled with practical instructions in *āsana* and *prāṇāyāma*, with an eye toward making the poses accessible and illuminating.

## Our Approach to Healing the Pelvic Floor

The information in this book comes from years of experience from two perspectives: hands-on clinical experience from the perspective of a pelvic health physical therapist, and guidance about yoga from the perspective of a Certified Iyengar Yoga Teacher. Throughout the text we have tried to be clear about when we are using language and ideas that are more clinical versus yogic. Of course, some overlap is inevitable, and we hope you will appreciate the connections (and differences) that we highlight between these two knowledge systems.

While we draw on both of these traditions, in some ways our approach to presenting the material and our approach to learning is not traditional. We encourage you to talk openly with fellow practitioners, teachers, pelvic health professionals, and trusted friends about the information presented here as well as about your own experiences and findings, as this will help you build your own subjective body of knowledge that is most helpful to you.

## Gender Inclusivity

We have experience in our courses working with people of many genders, and it is our intention that this book is inviting and accessible to anyone with a pelvis. Though the emphasis of this book is on birthing and the organs and anatomy that are associated with the ability to do so, we are committed to using anatomical language that is inclusive. Our approach is to find common language so that anyone can easily relate to the anatomy presented. We also recognize that there are a variety of differences and preferences when it comes to language, and not everyone agrees on each term. For example, we use the word vagina frequently in this book, but we also use the terms vaginal canal, vault, opening, and genitalia as well as sometimes describing the pelvis and pelvic floor without using any of these terms at all. We hope that our descriptions address a wide variety of people and experiences. Further, we believe that anyone can benefit from the exercises, āsanas, and prāṇāyāma included here, regardless of gender, and we've geared our instructions with that intention.

## How to Use This Book

This book is broken into three chapters: "Anatomy of the Pelvic Floor," "Sequences of Āsanas for Practice," and a chapter on "Special Topics." We encourage you to read chapter 1, "Anatomy of the Pelvic Floor," thoroughly before or at the same time as practicing the sequences given in chapter 2. Anatomy can be overwhelming to learn at first, but we have attempted to present the information with an eye toward experiencing and feeling these important parts of the body. We've included information about how to visualize, feel, and sense more subtle aspects of anatomy and breath, which is essential when practicing the āsanas. Additionally, we give information about pelvic floor neighbors like the muscles of the hips and abdomen that may help you better understand the interplay and interdependence of the incredible systems within your body.

Chapter 2 provides sequences of āsana and prāṇāyāma for practice. The poses in this book are based on the principles of Iyengar Yoga. We recommend that you initially follow the sequences in the order they are given as they describe a progressive arc of healing. The sequences can be roughly broken up into three phases that we feel are important for anyone working with pelvic floor symptoms, regardless of their condition or whether they are postpartum. The first stage focuses on relaxation and coordinated breathing. The second stage works on better alignment of the pelvis and the pelvic organs, and developing stability in the pelvic region. The third phase reflects a move toward strengthening the neighboring regions around the pelvis, including the legs, spine, and abdominal core. Once this general arc is understood, the information in the sequences can be adapted into a general yoga practice.

The sequences in chapter 2 have been intentionally kept simple, straightforward, and manageable even for beginners or those with limited time. Many students come to yoga for the first time after having a baby, and these students may easily feel overwhelmed with too much information, too many poses, or complicated setups. We have kept this in mind as we present the progression of sequences. Alternately, for those with more experience, or those with specific symptoms like hip or back pain, extra props may be needed to make a pose therapeutic and beneficial. There is no simple prescription or magic pose that will cure your symptoms; however, instructions are aimed at explaining the *how* and *why* of each pose, as well as the necessary *actions* of the pelvic floor, so that you can learn to feel in your own body the effects of the poses. More advanced practitioners may appreciate this, especially in going to a more advanced stage of a pose or a more prop-intensive setup. More experienced practitioners can also incorporate these short sequences easily into their regular practice. Any pose that causes pain should be avoided, and you can work with this book under the supervision of a local Certified Iyengar Yoga Teacher to optimize the therapeutic benefits of the poses.

We are indebted to the work of Geeta Iyengar, Rita Keller, and Kerstin Khattab in their book *Iyengar Yoga for Motherhood*, and you will notice some similarities to their approach. We have followed their general guidelines about the three postpartum trimesters, taking place roughly four to six weeks after birth and continuing through six to eight months. General timelines are given for when it is safe to start practicing certain poses after childbirth. Keep in mind that these are suggestions, and that each person's body and situation are different. We recommend that you work through this book progressively, even if you are months or years postpartum, or not postpartum at all. The presentation of the poses and the instructions is systematic, building on itself, and you may miss some essential building blocks if you skip ahead.

Chapter 3 presents some special topics and more detailed information about common pelvic floor and postpartum symptoms that students may experience. Again, we encourage you not to just jump to these as a prescription, but to work through the material sequentially, using the information in chapter 3 to augment your practice. We also encourage you to read through the entirety of chapter 3 even if you are not experiencing each specific symptom. As in many therapeutic approaches to āsana, what helps one person with one condition may also be helpful for someone experiencing a different condition, and in several sections we refer back to principles and actions within poses that can be helpful for a variety of practitioners. Teachers especially may want to familiarize themselves with these sections to better help their students.

The information in this book is not intended as medical advice, and you should always follow the advice of your doctor or health care provider. When in doubt, communicate with your providers or contact your local Certified Iyengar Yoga Teacher.

## Healing through the Kośas: Moving from Outer to Inner

Conventional modern medical anatomy differs in some important ways from yogic ideas of anatomy, and we draw on both traditions in this text. One concept that comes from yoga but can easily be applied to the anatomy of the pelvic floor is the idea of kośas. The Sanskrit word *kośa* translates to layer or sheath. In yoga, there are five kośas of the body that move from outer or more gross to inner or more subtle, representing five layers of experience in the body. You might visualize an onion with its many layers, each layer peeled away to reveal the layer underneath. The five layers of the body are *annamaya kośa* or physical body, *prāṇamaya kośa* or breath or energy body, *manomaya kośa* or mental body, *vijñānamaya kośa* or wisdom body, and *ānandamaya kośa* or bliss body.

Yoga students are well aware that in learning about their own bodies, insights can be experienced at any of these five layers. When first starting out on your yoga anatomy journey, it may be helpful to observe and understand the physical body for some time. As we learn about the pelvis, we need to familiarize ourselves with the bones, joints, and muscles of the pelvis. However, the pelvis is a highly sensitive, meaningful, and unconscious part of our own anatomy. Even learning about the muscles, which are deeply internal, can bring us into a profound inner experience. As we explore inside the pelvis, we may notice that our breathing changes or we have energetic reactions. Mental reactions, both positive and negative, may also be felt. As we understand more about our own anatomy and can connect more deeply to this part of the body, we may find we gain consciousness, awareness, and understanding where we did not previously experience it. Finally, we may experience healing and integration, which can bring deep comfort, joy, and even bliss.

It may be helpful for you to keep this image of the onion and its many layers in mind as you proceed, understanding that the journey may take some time. We hope that your pelvic floor journey is meaningful, and we are honored to be going on this adventure together.

# ANATOMY *of the* PELVIC FLOOR

I n this chapter we discuss the anatomy of the pelvis and other surrounding regions with a focus on how to experientially feel these areas in your own body. While we may use clinical language at times, it is helpful not just to memorize this information in your head but to take time to visualize, feel, and sense the bones, joints, muscles, and organs that make up your pelvis. This will help you better absorb and apply the anatomical information and can profoundly deepen your practice of yoga as well as your daily movements. This felt knowledge can also be empowering, especially when searching for help with a specific problem or set of symptoms, aiding you in your understanding and communication about the issue. Having a deeper understanding of your own anatomy can help you cope with uncertainty or fear if you are experiencing something painful or new to you, especially in the postpartum recovery period.

The language used in this book focuses on the anatomy typically associated with birthing, and we use the terms vagina, clitoris, vaginal canal, and uterus frequently. We have made every attempt to describe these areas *without* ascribing gender, and we welcome you to substitute any other terms that may help you have a deeper connection to your own body, such as external gonads, genital opening, vault, front hole, middle hole, and so on. Further, many of the muscles of the pelvic floor are common to all, no matter your gender, and the instructions for accessing the pelvic floor muscles will not differ from those given here. We hope that our approach to presenting the information helps you develop a deeper, more knowledgeable, and more loving connection to your own body.

## Bony Anatomy of the Pelvis

The pelvis is the central point in the human body, and it can be a source of great pleasure and pain, at once mysterious and illuminating. Pelvises come in all shapes and sizes. The pelvis is a wonder as it is sturdy and provides stability and steadiness to the body, but it also houses a changing environment within. Among its many functions, the pelvis houses and supports organs, eliminates waste, allows for reproduction, and supports weight transfer and movement throughout the body.

As we explore and orient ourselves to the pelvis, take a moment to familiarize yourself with the four anatomical planes that run through the body so that you can appreciate and visualize multidimensional connections and relationships between the body's various structures. The sagittal plane separates the left and right sides of the body, and the frontal plane separates the front and back of the body. The transverse plane runs horizontally and the oblique plane runs at diagonal angles through the body. As you read through chapter 1, we encourage the use of any tools that aid your individual learning process, including imagination, visualization, touch, illustrations, or the use of 3-D models.

As we dive into pelvic anatomy, note the overall shape of the pelvis, with its contours and curves; there is almost no area of the pelvis that is straight or linear in form. The pelvis is formed by a pair of pelvic bones made up of three distinct bones—the ilium, ischium, and pubis—that fuse in adolescence or early adulthood.[1] Orient yourself to the front view of the pelvis (Figure 1.1). With your hands, feel just below your waist for the top of the ilium. Beneath this bony shelf the ilium becomes broad and fan-shaped. Move your hands to the front surface of the ilium and feel for the "headlights" of the pelvis, the anterior superior iliac spine. Move your hands down the front and center of the pelvis and gently feel your pubic bone on each side. Take a moment to appreciate the height of this bone. In between each pubic bone is a space called the pubic symphysis. Within this space is a disc that allows for force absorption and movement of the pelvis during childbirth. Continuing from the bottom of the pubic bone, follow the diagonal line laterally and posteriorly, down and out to the side and back, toward the curved surface of the ischial bone. Here we come to the ischial tuberosities, commonly referred to as buttock or "sitz" bones. Notice the transition from the thin, flat pubic bone to the wide, rounded ischial bones that mark the bottom, or inferior aspect, of the pelvis. Continue to follow this up the back of the pelvis to meet the posterior aspect of the ilium and the inferior aspect of the hip joint (Figure 1.2).

To clearly locate the hip joint, find the large, round head of the femur bone where it meets the concave surface of the acetabulum. Deep within this surface is where the three distinct pelvic bones described above meet to create a ball-and-socket joint, the femoroacetabular or hip joint. Return to the posterior inferior aspect of the hip joint. As we seek the bony projection of the ischial spine on each side of the pelvis, imagine that you can move medially toward the inner framework of your pelvis to locate them. Since these projections are located deeply within the pelvic bowl, it's difficult to feel them on your own body. You may find it helpful to refer to the images of the bony pelvis to view these important landmarks.

Return to the back of the pelvis and, feeling with your hands or following with the images, notice the top, thin, flat surface of the ilium. As this bone descends toward the midline, it hugs each side of the sacrum. The sacrum is made up of

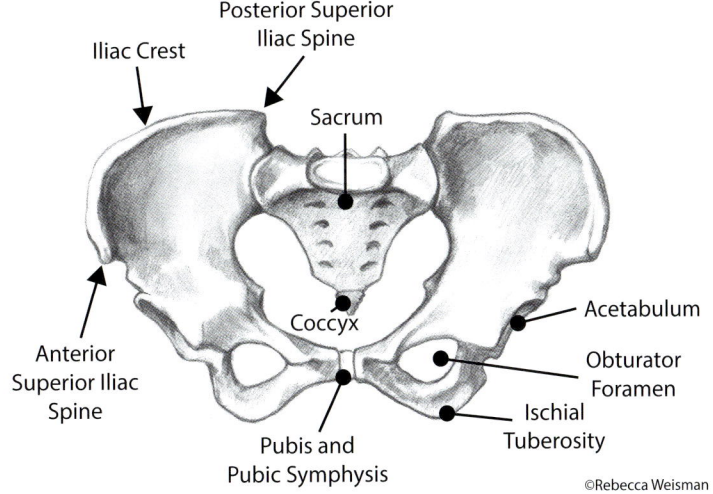

FIGURE 1.1.  **Anterior view of the pelvis**

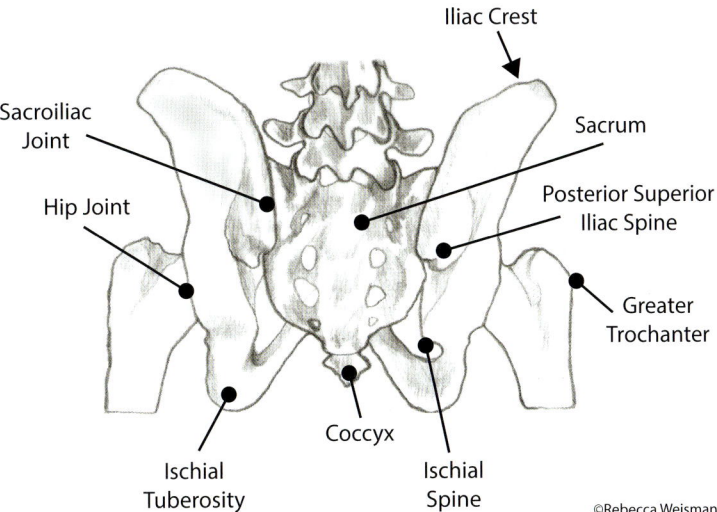

FIGURE 1.2.  **Posterior view of the bony pelvis**

four or five smaller bones that are fused to form one large, curved bone. Cup your hand as if holding water in your palm to gain an idea of the shape and size of the sacrum. The top of the sacrum meets the lumbar spine at the lumbosacral joint. It bridges the left and right sides of the pelvis via the sacroiliac joint, where a few degrees of motion are available in all planes. The depth and length of the sacroiliac joint can be seen in the illustrations here from the front and back of the pelvis, where it's reinforced by a large network of strong ligaments, including the sacrotuberous and sacrospinous ligaments. Large holes called the sacral foramina can be seen on each side of the sacrum along its entire length. These holes are where nerves and vessels exit the spine to reach the rest of the body.

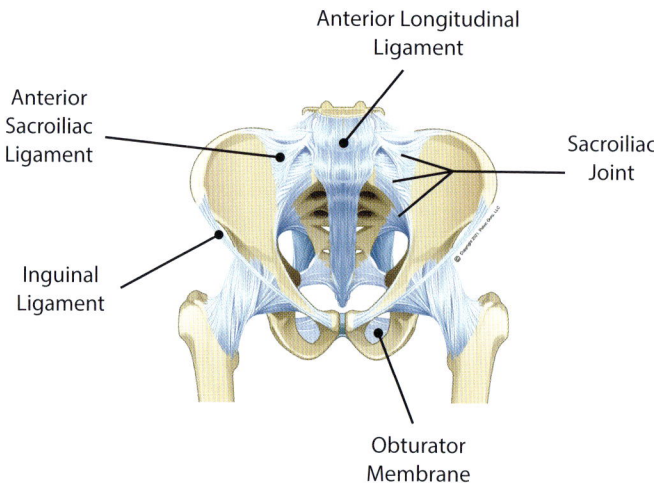

**FIGURE 1.3.** Pelvic ligaments, anterior view

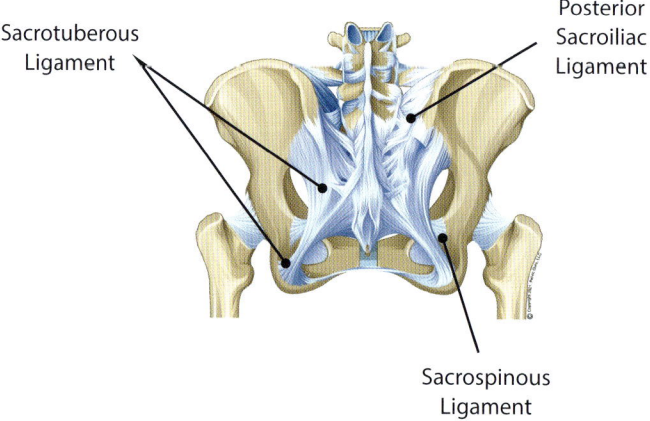

**FIGURE 1.4.** Pelvic ligaments, posterior view

Below the sacroiliac joint, the bottom third of the sacrum connects with another fused set of bones to form the coccyx, also known as the tailbone. The space between the sacrum and coccyx form the sacrococcygeal joint, where a small degree of motion is available in all planes. This area is reinforced by many of the same ligaments that are found at the lumbosacral and sacroiliac joints above. In figure 1.4, notice how many ligaments overlap the sacrum, pelvis, and lower spine, creating a network of support. They run along the entire front and back lengths of the spinal column (anterior and posterior longitudinal spinal ligament), from the sacrum to the buttock bones (sacrotuberous ligament), from the sacrum to the spine (sacrospinal ligament), from the sacrum to the coccyx (sacrococcygeal ligament), from the sacrum to the ilium (sacroiliac ligament), and from the ilium to the spine (iliolumbar ligament).

These ligaments are incredibly important because they are the primary means of support for the pelvis and provide attachment sites for some muscles that further reinforce the pelvis. Throughout pregnancy and specifically during labor and delivery, the length, support, and structure provided by these ligaments changes to allow space for growth, broadening and eventually opening to allow for movement of the baby out of the pelvis. After birth, the ligaments often remain lengthened since ligaments aren't elastic in the same way as muscle tissue; they generally don't rebound as efficiently or as completely on their own. This can create instability in the pelvis. Specific attention to returning to your optimal alignment and learning to utilize the pelvic floor muscles as well as the hip muscles to stabilize the pelvis can be very helpful, as we discuss throughout this text.

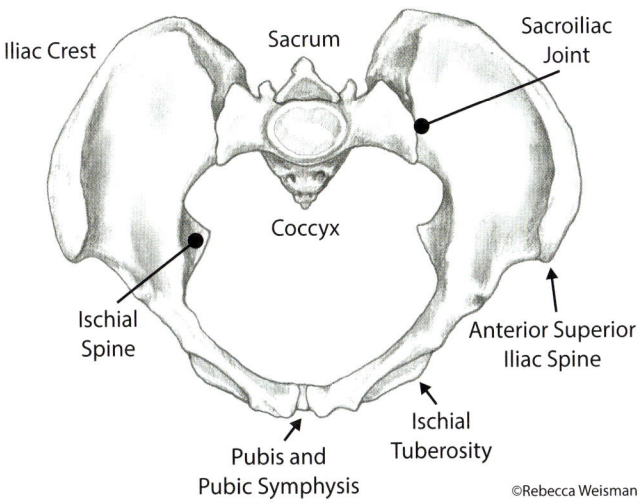

©Rebecca Weisman

FIGURE 1.5.  Superior view of the pelvis

Now that you've explored the outer structure and landmarks of the pelvis, it's equally important to recognize the inner bony landmarks that demarcate the pelvic inlet and outlet. The size and shape of the pelvic inlet and outlet vary greatly among people based on the overall shape of each individual pelvis. Some pelvises are tall and narrow while others tend to be shorter and wider, providing more space for the processes of pregnancy and childbirth.

Utilizing the illustration of the superior (top) view of the Bony Pelvis (fig. 1.5), look down into the pelvis from above. The bony borders of the pelvis include the top of the sacrum, inner ilium, and pubic bones. This wide, irregularly shaped oval space is the pelvic inlet. During pregnancy, the pelvic inlet is the entrance to the birth canal. In some individuals it holds space for parts of the lower intestines and ureters, tubes that transport urine from the kidneys to the bladder.

Shift your perspective and look at the bony pelvis from below (fig. 1.6). The circumference of this irregularly shaped oval, made up of the borders of the pubic and ischial bones and coccyx, outlines the pelvic outlet. The pelvic outlet houses the urinary bladder, internal reproductive organs, and colon. Familiarizing yourself with the various boundaries, landmarks, and spaces within the pelvis helps to deepen your appreciation of how these pieces fit together, especially as we explore the interplay of these parts in the chapters ahead.

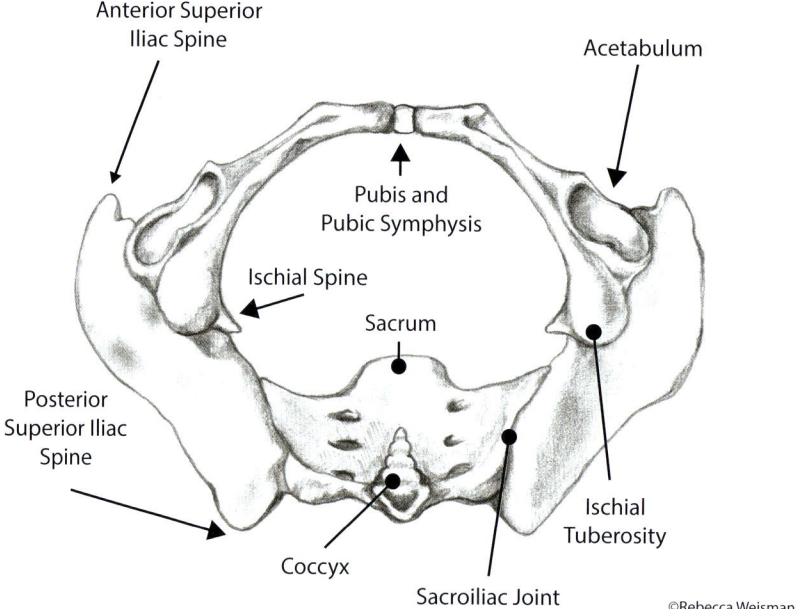

©Rebecca Weisman

**FIGURE 1.6. Inferior view of the bony pelvis**

# Pelvic Floor Muscles

As we explore deeper into the pelvis, we arrive at the pelvic floor muscles (PFMs), surrounded by a layer of fascial tissue. Fascia is found throughout the body as a thin, uninterrupted layer of elastic tissue that forms a fluid matrix that surrounds and penetrates all structures of the body from head to toe. While detecting fascia in an illustration or even through touch can be difficult, fascia informs all our movement patterns seen on the outside and felt within.

Inside the fascia we encounter the pelvic floor muscles. These are most commonly recognized as three distinct layers of tissue interconnected by fasciae that attach to the bony pelvis and other strong connective tissues within the pelvis. Sometimes seen as a muscular sling, these layers form a diamond shape, overlapping and extending in many directions, and they bridge the space between the pelvic bones. The multidirectional connections within each layer of muscle reinforce pelvic support for your organs and their functions, and they create depth to form a container, the pelvic bowl. While often referred to as a bowl or hammock, in living bodies the pelvic floor muscles actually dome slightly upward in their resting position. As you begin to visualize the contents of your pelvic bowl, including your pelvic organs, you might imagine these contents resting atop a domed structure rather than slumping down into a hammock. The effect is quite different!

## MUSCLE TENSION AND MUSCLE TONE

Muscle tension is the force generated by a contraction of a muscle against any load. Sometimes the tension generated may be enough to move or change the position of the load by either lengthening or shortening the muscle fibers. This is known as an isotonic muscle contraction and is either concentric and shortening (for example, when bending your elbow, your bicep muscle shortens concentrically), or eccentric and lengthening (for example, when straightening your elbow, your bicep muscle lengthens eccentrically). Sometimes the tension generated is equal to the applied resistance, resulting in a static isometric contraction.

Muscle tone is the tension of a muscle when it is at rest and is not a reflection of muscle strength. Every body possesses a different resting or baseline level of tone. Changes in tone are typical and are necessary to support both movement and rest.[2] Tone exists on a spectrum and can influence changes in tension. Resting tension can be high or low, and in the pelvic floor muscles it is possible to have mixed levels of tension, meaning that one side of the pelvis or one group of muscles has high tension whereas a different part of the pelvis presents with lower tension. When considering your pelvic floor, it's important to develop an understanding of your own muscle qualities and degree of tension because it influences the overall health and function of your pelvis.

Some common physical symptoms that are associated with elevated pelvic tension are:

- generalized pelvic pain
- painful intercourse or pain with penetration
- difficulty with elimination
- urinary incontinence or frequency
- gastrointestinal issues
- organ prolapse

Some common physical symptoms associated with reduced pelvic tension include:

- urinary or bowel incontinence
- organ prolapse
- vaginal flatulence (air passing through the vagina)
- decreased overall sensation or connection with the pelvis

Your nervous system helps regulate your muscle tension by sending signals from the brain to the nerves, telling the muscles to contract or relax. It is because of this connection that tension can be influenced by both internal and external factors. For example, when the brain experiences a feeling, sensation, sound, thought, or movement that it perceives as a threat, signals related to threat (protectiveness, fear, anxiety, shallow breathing) are produced and sent out to the body. Conversely, experiences that are perceived as peaceful or restful signal relaxation in the body. Breathing and yoga practices help us experience this connection between our brain and our muscular patterns, and can help bring balance between them. As we discuss more in chapters 2 and 3, addressing high tension in the pelvic floor muscles is imperative as the muscles should learn to relax and lengthen in order to eventually contract efficiently. In other words, relaxation before strengthening!

Viewing the pelvis from below (fig. 1.7), trace the outline of the diamond shape of the first layer of pelvic floor muscles. Draw a horizontal line from one ischial tuberosity to the other so that you see two triangles within the diamond. The anterior or front urogenital triangle contains the genitals and urethra and their openings, and the posterior or back anal triangle contains the anus. The illustration shown here depicts a pelvis with a vagina. Notice that in between the vaginal opening and the anus at the midline of the body is a fibromuscular structure called the perineal body, sometimes referred to as the central tendon of the perineum, which is common to all pelvises, and separates the front and back triangles.

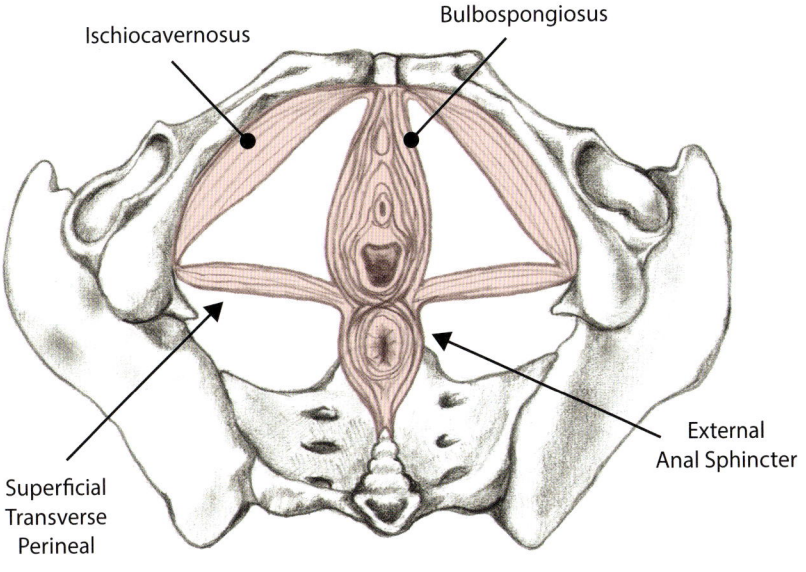

Ischiocavernosus

Bulbospongiosus

External
Anal Sphincter

Superficial
Transverse
Perineal

©Rebecca Weisman

**FIGURE 1.7. The first layer of pelvic floor muscles, inferior view**

The most superficial layer of pelvic floor muscles is made up of bulbocavernosus or bulbospongiosus, ischiocavernosus, superficial transverse perineal, and the external anal sphincter. While these muscles each have different attachments, all but the ischiocavernosus muscle attach at the center of the perineum. Each side of the ischiocavernosus muscle attaches at the clitoris and its respective ischial tuberosity (IT). From the IT, the superficial transverse perineal runs horizontally toward the center of the perineum on either side. Note that these two muscles, superficial transverse perineal and ischiocavernosus on each side, outline the urogenital triangle.

The bulbospongiosus forms a figure eight shape around the genital openings and sphincters. Viewing figure 1.7, from the center of the perineum, begin to trace one loop of a figure eight moving up and around the vaginal and urethral opening on one side, over the top of the clitoris and down the other side, back to the perineal body. Now cross over the perineal body and trace another loop around the anus, moving toward the tailbone on one side, returning up the other side to the perineal body. This loop traces the external anal sphincter, and your figure eight is complete. By tracing these shapes, you may begin to appreciate how the fibers of these muscles move in such a way as to reinforce one other at this most superficial layer. Indeed, these muscles play an important role in sphincter control (muscles relaxing or tightening to open or close openings and passages) and sexual function. Tension, pain, or weakness in this layer may influence these functions, as we discuss further in chapters 2 and 3. Visualizing these shapes may also give you more feeling and control at this layer, and help you understand how they influence the deeper layers.

Tables 1-3 outline the various pelvic floor muscles, their function, and their nerve innervation. This information may be useful if you are experiencing pain or other symptoms to help identify at which layer the pain is occurring. Additionally, you will note that the pelvic floor muscles are all innervated by the pudendal nerve and its branches, a peripheral nerve that arises from sacral nerve roots S2, S3, and S4. We further discuss the pudendal nerve and possible symptoms that may arise with its involvement in our discussion of the hip and gluteal muscles later in this chapter.

Immediately deep to the first layer of pelvic floor muscles is the perineal membrane. This is a thin layer of dense fascia that covers the urogenital and anal triangles and acts as a strong support for the pelvic organs and is an attachment site for the bulbocavernosus and ischiocavernosus muscles in layer 1. Located within the layer of the perineal membrane is an opening called

TABLE 1:  Layer 1 pelvic floor muscles in a pelvis with a vagina[3]

| MUSCLE | ACTION | NERVE INNERVATION |
|---|---|---|
| bulbocavernosus/ bulbospongiosus | assists in erection of the clitoris and bulb of the clitoral vestibule; supports the perineal body | pudendal nerve |
| ischiocavernosus | pushes blood from the root of the clitoris to the body to maintain erection during sexual arousal | pudendal nerve |
| superficial transverse perineal | constricts the urethra and vagina; helps to maintain urinary continence | pudendal nerve |
| external anal sphincter | provides voluntary control of defecation by remaining in a tonic state until ready to empty | pudendal nerve |

the urogenital hiatus, which accommodates the rectum, the end of the gastrointestinal system posteriorly, and the vagina and urethra anteriorly.

Just beyond the perineal membrane is layer 2 of the pelvic floor muscles. This layer consists of the deep transverse perineal muscle, external urethral

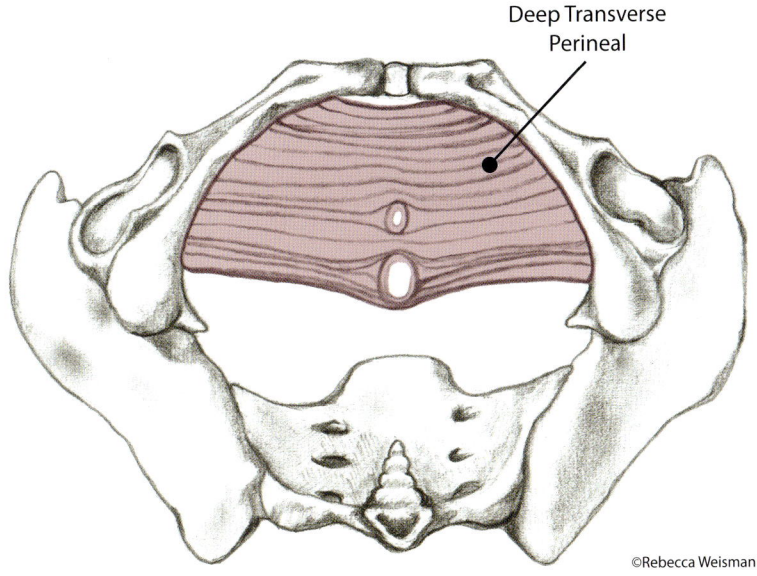

Deep Transverse
Perineal

©Rebecca Weisman

FIGURE 1.8.  Second layer of pelvic floor muscles, inferior view

sphincter, compressor urethrae, and sphincter urethrovaginalis, which constrict the urethra and vagina to aid in urinary continence. The deep transverse perineal muscle has horizontally oriented muscle fibers throughout the urogenital triangle, while the sphincter and compressor muscles are oriented more vertically, surrounding the circumference of the vaginal and urethral openings.[4] Imagine these muscle fiber orientations in your own body and the directions they move when they contract, release, or expand. Often there can be weakness or tension at the perineal body and difficulty contracting, releasing, or isolating movement here. This layer is especially relevant when urinary symptoms are present, as we discuss further in chapter 3.

The deepest layer of the pelvic floor muscles is layer 3, also referred to as the pelvic diaphragm. While the first two layers can be viewed from the outside looking in, if we change our perspective and look into the pelvic bowl from above, we can view the third layer of pelvic floor muscles. This layer, which lines the inner framework of the lower pelvic bones, gives shape to the bottom of the pelvis and comes into immediate contact with the pelvic organs, supporting them from below. The muscles that make up this deepest layer are ischiococcygeus, which flexes the tailbone and aids in urination and defecation, and puborectalis, pubococcygeus, and iliococcygeus which together are called the levator ani group of muscles.

**TABLE 2:** Layer 2 pelvic floor muscles in a pelvis with a vagina

| MUSCLE | ACTION | INNERVATION |
| --- | --- | --- |
| deep transverse perineal | fixation of the perineal body (central tendon of perineum); support of the pelvic floor; expulsion of last drops of urine | perineal branch of pudendal nerve |
| external urethral sphincter | maintains urinary continence; constricts vaginal canal | perineal branch of pudendal nerve |
| compressor urethrae | controls urination and maintains urinary continence by compressing the urethra | perineal branch of pudendal nerve |
| sphincter urethrovaginalis | controls urination | perineal branch of pudendal nerve |

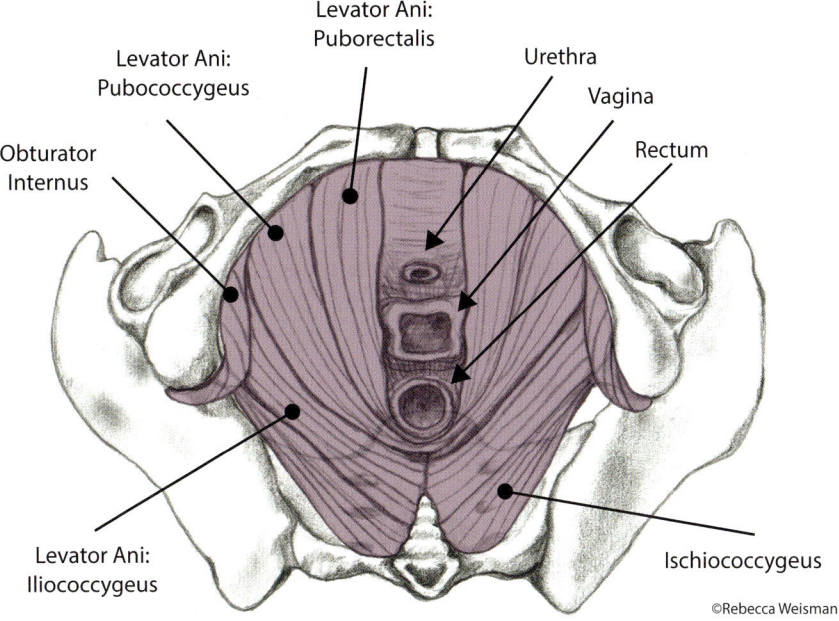

Levator Ani:
Puborectalis

Levator Ani:
Pubococcygeus

Urethra

Vagina

Rectum

Obturator
Internus

Levator Ani:
Iliococcygeus

Ischiococcygeus

©Rebecca Weisman

**FIGURE 1.9.** Third layer of pelvic floor muscles, inferior view

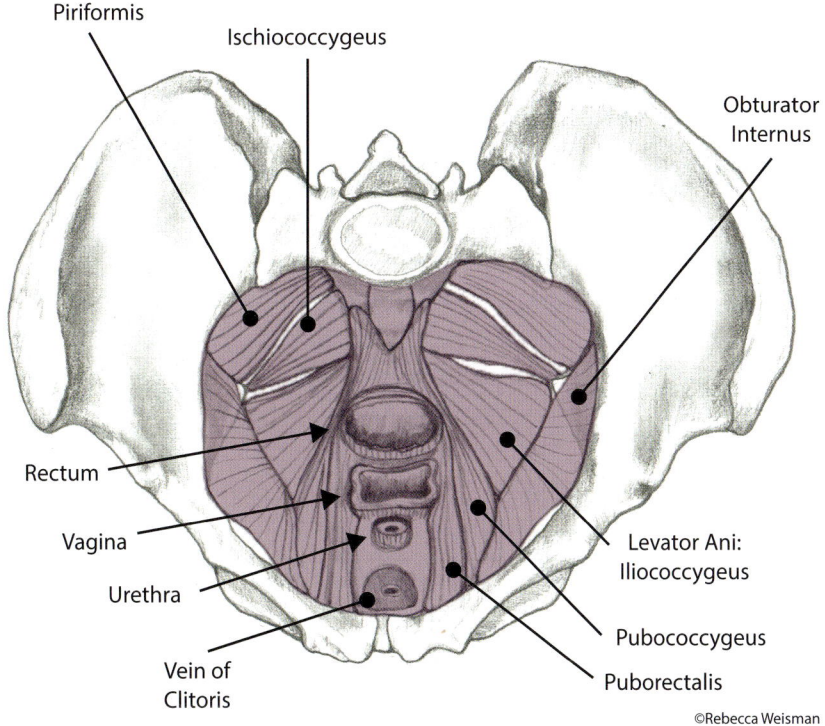

Piriformis

Ischiococcygeus

Obturator
Internus

Rectum

Vagina

Urethra

Levator Ani:
Iliococcygeus

Pubococcygeus

Puborectalis

Vein of
Clitoris

©Rebecca Weisman

**FIGURE 1.10.** Third layer of pelvic floor muscles, superior view

The levator ani muscles span a substantial portion of the pelvic floor. The main function of the levator ani is to provide muscular support and stability to the abdominal and pelvic viscera and to resist increases in intra-abdominal pressure. Weakness in this layer may hinder the functioning and alignment of the organs. Without these muscles, the abdominal and pelvic organs would drop straight out of your abdomen and pelvis! While each individual is different, tension in the levator ani muscles may be felt as deep, achy pain and may be connected to pain in neighboring areas such as the lower back, sacrum, and hip. The levator ani muscles also support sexual function, defecation, and urination, and they control opening and closing of the levator hiatus.

From an external perspective (fig 1.9), notice the direction of the third layer muscle fibers running anterior-posterior or front-back across the depth of the pelvic bowl. Now look into the bowl (fig 1.10) and you will see a similar pattern at the immediate center of the pelvis. As you follow the muscles laterally, notice that the direction of the muscle fibers shift diagonally, oriented toward the sides of the pelvic bowl. The multilayered and multidirectional arrangement of the layers of pelvic floor muscle and tissue act to reinforce and support the contents of the bowl.

**TABLE 3:** Layer 3 pelvic floor muscles in a pelvis with a vagina

| MUSCLE | ACTION | INNERVATION |
|---|---|---|
| puborectalis | forms a sling around the lower rectum; acts in association with the internal and external anal sphincter in the process of defecation | S3, S4 (nerve to levator ani), pudendal nerve |
| pubococcygeus | supports the vagina; aids ejaculation and orgasm; assists in proper positioning of the fetus head | S3, S4 (nerve to levator ani), pudendal nerve |
| iliococcygeus | provides a secure anchoring point for the pelvic floor, forms the midline raphe after it meets the fibers from the opposite side | S4, pudendal nerve |
| coccygeus/ ischiococcygeus | supports the pelvic viscera; flexes the coccyx; aids the puborectalis to control urination and defecation | S4, S5 |

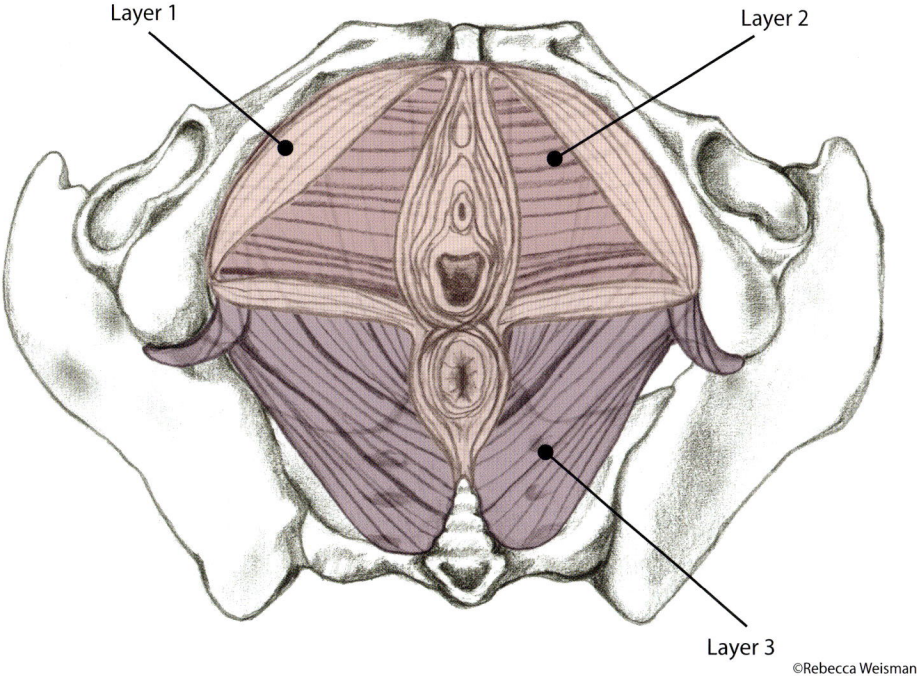

Layer 1

Layer 2

Layer 3

©Rebecca Weisman

FIGURE 1.11. **All three layers of pelvic floor muscles, inferior view**

## DOING A PELVIC SELF-ASSESSMENT

A self-assessment can be a helpful and empowering tool for those who want to better understand and connect with their own muscular anatomy. Observing and feeling your unique pelvic anatomy helps establish a baseline familiarity with your external and internal landscape and can help you gather information related to strength and relaxation, tone, coordination, and pain. This section has instructions for doing a self-assessment, either vaginally or rectally.

If you are experiencing active bleeding due to menstruation or birth, wait until the bleeding has completely stopped and you are fully healed. Postpartum individuals should wait until you have clearance from your provider, approximately four to six weeks postpartum. If you already know that touch around the vagina or vulva or penetration vaginally is painful, begin with visualizing a self-assessment, following the cues given here. Working directly with a pelvic physical therapist is recommended.

Once you've determined that you're ready to begin, thoroughly wash your hands with soap and water. Arrange your space so that it is quiet and private. Find a comfortable semi-reclined position. You may want to lean your back against a wall or headboard and have some pillows nearby to support your body. It may be helpful to have a notebook and pen nearby to record any observations or questions that arise.

## External Observations

1. Hold a hand mirror and separate your legs so that you can see your external pelvis in the mirror.

2. Look at your perineum between the anus and genitals and gently press this area with one finger. Does it bounce? Is it stiff or firm?

3. Separate your labia and look at your vaginal opening. Alternatively, you can separate your buttocks and look at the anus if you are doing the assessment rectally. Squeeze and hold the muscles around your vaginal opening or anus and notice what happens when you engage the muscles around this area. Do you see any movement or change in shape? If so, how much movement do you see, and in which direction?

4. Let go of your muscle squeeze and rest. Now, gently bear down. Maintain this position for a few seconds and note whether you see any movement or change in shape. If so, how much, and in which direction?

## Internal Observations

### Internal Vaginal Assessment

1. First, wash your hands with soap and water. For the internal vaginal assessment, you may want to use a small amount of oil (coconut or olive) or a water-based lubricant to help your fingers slide and glide more comfortably over your tissue.

2. It can be helpful to imagine the opening of the vagina as an elongated clock. From your position and orientation, the top of the clock, 12 o'clock, is just beneath the clitoris. The bottom of the clock, 6 o'clock, is straight down toward the perineum. From the center of your vagina, draw an imaginary straight line to the left side of the vaginal opening and find the 3 o'clock position. Return to center, move straight across to the right side, and find 9 o'clock.

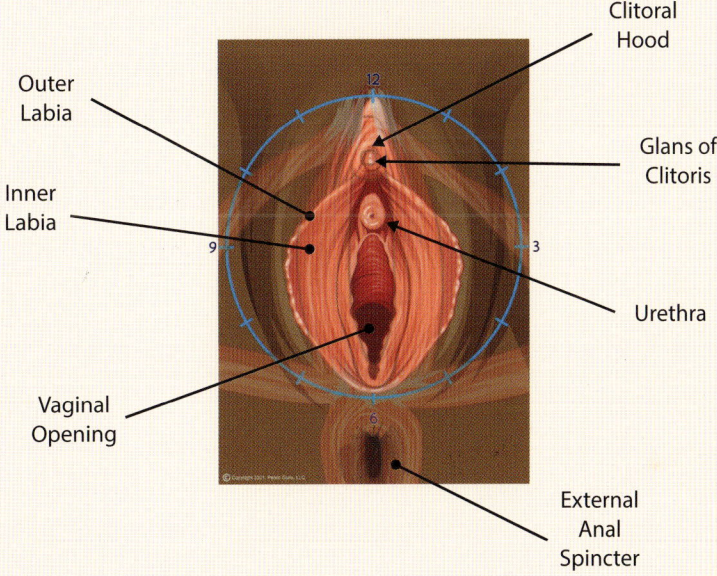

**FIGURE 1.12.  Vulvar clock**

3. Feel one side of the vagina at a time using the thumb opposite of the side you're working on. Keep in mind that you are feeling for muscle tissue, so don't apply pressure internally near the 12 and 6 o'clock positions, as this is where your bladder and rectum are positioned.

4. Insert your right thumb gradually, beginning with your thumbnail, then up to the first knuckle and perhaps eventually to the base of your thumb. Lightly sweep your right thumb along the side wall of

the pelvis, between the 1 o'clock and 5 o'clock positions. Note the quality of the tissue you feel, any pain or tenderness, and temperature or sensory changes. If you observe any places of notable pain or trigger points, stay for a few breaths, lightly pressing the area, and focus on releasing with the inhalation.

5.  When you're finished on that side, remove your thumb and repeat the entire process on the opposite side using your left thumb to feel between 7 o'clock and 11 o'clock.

6.  Notice and record any differences between the two sides.

7.  After you've completed sweeping on both sides, insert one or two fingers straight into the vaginal opening and gently contract your pelvic floor muscles. Consider the following:

    a.  How long can you hold the muscle contraction before the muscles let go?

    b.  Can you feel the muscles engage around your finger?

    c.  When you engage your muscles, do you detect a lift of your finger inward?

8.  Let go of the muscle contraction. Notice whether you are able to let go immediately and completely.

9.  Next, gently bear down. Maintain this action for a few seconds and note whether you feel your finger move in a particular direction. It should feel like it moves out slightly.

10. Remove your finger completely and wash your hands with soap and water.

### Internal Rectal Assessment

Performing a rectal assessment is another way to feel some of the pelvic floor muscles, but because the anal sphincters hold a lot of natural tension, you may not be able to go as deep or feel as much. Doing a rectal assessment can also be helpful if you are experiencing tailbone pain, and if muscle tension is found, using a pelvic wand can be very effective in releasing trigger points. (A pelvic wand can also be used for a vaginal assessment and release following the same instructions above.) For more about using a pelvic wand, see the "Additional Resources" appendix.

1. Begin by washing your hands with soap and water. Lie on your side with your bottom leg straight and your top leg bent at your knee and hip and supported on a stack of pillows.

2. Imagine the face of a clock. The top of the clock, 12 o'clock, is facing the pubic bone, and 6 o'clock is toward the bottom near the tailbone or coccyx.

3. Use lubricant (olive oil, coconut oil, or a water-based lubricant) and place gentle pressure around the anus for about thirty seconds until it softens and relaxes. This will be more noticeable if there's elevated tone or tension. Work with a soft breath and use your inhalation to release tension.

4. Insert your lubricated or gloved index finger into your rectum up to your first knuckle, about half an inch inside. Beginning at 1 o'clock, barely inside the anus, apply very gentle pressure and move around the clock, noting what you feel. You may need to alternate your position, changing which side you are lying on, in order to feel the deeper pelvic muscles.

5. Make your way around the clock. Skip the very bottom of the clock and the very top of the clock, as this is your tailbone and your prostate area or bladder, respectively. Remember to stay connected with your breath!

6. To get a sense of strength and coordination, squeeze your muscles around your finger. Can you do this? If so, how long can you hold?

7. Release your contraction. Are you able to do this completely? Do you feel any change in tension around your finger?

8. Now bear down and maintain this position for a few seconds. Are you able to bear down effectively? What direction do you feel your finger move? Do you notice a change in sensation?

9. From a side-lying position, reach your finger toward your tail-bone or feel for the muscles surrounding it. You'll know you're in the right area if you feel an increase in pressure or sensation in this region. If you feel an area of elevated tension, main-tain a comfortable amount of pressure and a few cycles of breath, focusing on your inhale to help release tension further. This can also be done in a prone position, as in Adho Mukha Vīrāsana, which may allow you to feel the tailbone more easily.

10. When you're finished, remove your finger completely and wash your hands with soap and water.

Once you've finished, acknowledge the work you and your body have done just by showing up. Thank your body and yourself for this vulner-able and important inquiry.

## Pelvic Organs

Following the pelvic anatomy closer to center, we arrive at the pelvic organs. The pelvic organs include the bladder and rectum, and for some people the uterus, ovaries, cervix, vagina, uterine tubes, clitoris, penis, prostate, or testicles. Take a moment to appreciate how the sacrum in back and the pubic bone in front create an external cradle of support for the organs. Many changes take place within this space on a daily basis and over your lifetime, including changes in

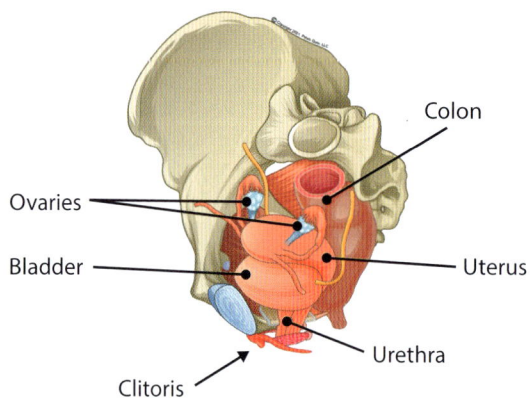

FIGURE 1.13. **Pelvic organs**

size and volume that occur due to natural processes such as urination and defecation, arousal, menstruation, pregnancy, and menopause.

Some organs like the bladder, uterus, and rectum are nestled closely together and give support to one another simply by being there. When a volume change occurs with one of these organs, it can affect the others. Likewise, if one or more organs change position or are removed, it can affect the support, position, and even function of the others. As organs change in size, shape, and position, they need continued support. This is provided through fascial, muscular, and an impressive network of ligamentous connections that allow for a balance of stability and movement.

## Bladder

The bladder is positioned behind the pubic bone and in front of the uterus. It's a hollow, membranous sac, somewhat triangular shaped, composed of smooth involuntary muscle fibers interwoven in multiple different directions, collectively known as the detrusor muscle. The orientation of the detrusor muscle fibers helps the bladder adapt in shape and size, allowing it to relax while it collects urine descending from the kidneys and ureters above. With urination, the detrusor muscle contracts to move urine out of the bladder and into the urethra. Here, the internal urethral sphincter regulates involuntary urine flow from the bladder to the urethra, while the external urethral sphincter allows for voluntary control of the urine from the bladder to the urethra. It's supported by the pubic bone, uterus, pelvic muscles, and various ligamentous connections on its anterior, lateral, posterior, and superior surfaces.

Due to its position in the pelvis and relationship to other organs, as the fetus and uterus grow during pregnancy, the bladder and urethra can become compressed forward and downward, and the amount of urine it holds may be reduced. Further, the tension of the pelvic floor muscles can affect the function of the bladder, as they are closely connected, which we explore in more detail in chapter 3.

## Uterus

The uterus is shaped like an upside-down pear. It is positioned between the bladder in front and the rectum in back. Fanning off this central organ from each side near its top are the uterine tubes and ovaries. There are a number of strong ligaments that support these organs, including the round, uterosacral, broad, and ovarian ligaments. Extending from the bottom of the uterus is the cervix, a narrow pathway that bridges the uterus and the vaginal canal. The

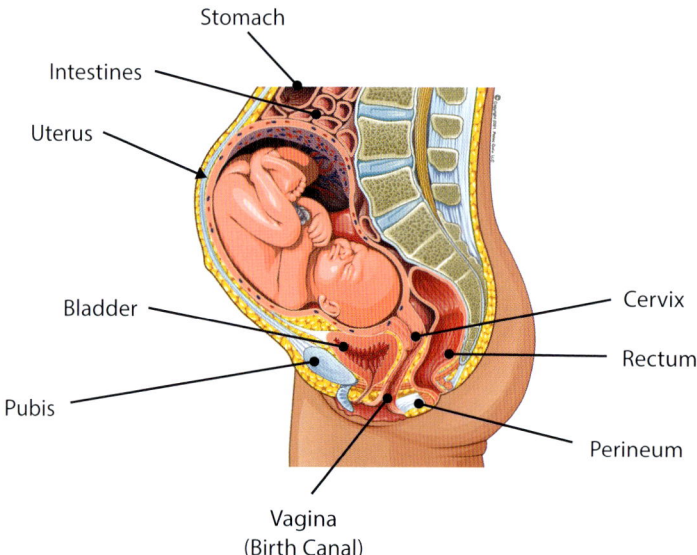

**FIGURE 1.14.** **Late-term gestation with fetus**

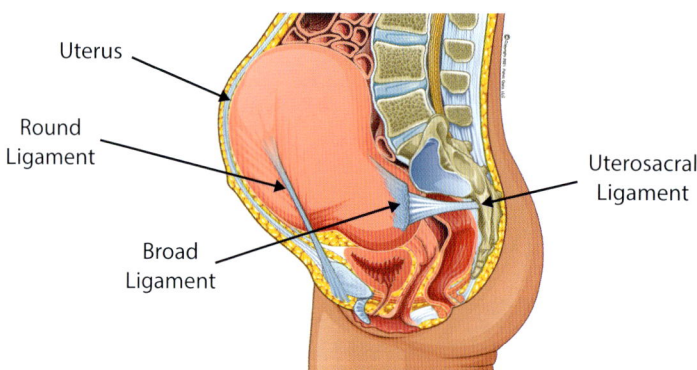

**FIGURE 1.15.** **Late-term gestation with uterus**

vaginal canal, sometimes referred to as the birth canal, is lined with muscle and extends to the outside of the body.

Various processes and events can affect the size and shape of the uterus, sometimes occupying more space, and at other times, less space. Pregnancy is a notable example of an increase in size and shape, so much so that during the third trimester, the uterus can stretch to the size of a watermelon! Consider the influences a change like this could have on surrounding organs and structures, such as changes of position of the organs and tension changes in muscles, ligaments, and supporting structures.

## Clitoris

The clitoris is an organ with most of its anatomy located internally. Only a small portion, the glans clitoris and clitoral hood, are visible externally. The glans, what most people refer to as the clitoris, is located just above the urethra. It is roughly pea size and contains a high concentration of nerve endings, making it extremely sensitive to touch. The clitoral hood surrounds the glans and is formed by the connection of the two sides of the labia minora. Clitoral hood size and degree of coverage vary from person to person.

Connected to the glans internally is the body of the clitoris. It extends upward into the pelvis and attaches to the pubic bone via ligamentous attachments that help it maintain its forward bent position. From the body, the clitoris divides in half to form the paired crura, which can be thought of as the legs of the clitoris, and vestibular bulbs. The bulbs extend through and behind the labia, urethra, and vaginal canal and toward the anus. These structures contain erectile tissue that swells with blood during sexual arousal and increases lubrication in the vagina.

Due to a high concentration of nerve endings, the clitoris is one of many erogenous zones in the body, meaning stimulation of this area can cause a physiologic response that results in sexual arousal.[5] For people who have a clitoris, it is one of the primary sources of sexual pleasure. Orgasms most commonly come from stimulation of the clitoris, which can be directly on the glans, internally, or through stimulation of other parts of the vulva.[6]

During the postpartum period, some people experience clitoral pain. This could be related to a condition called pubic symphysis dysfunction, a separation of the pubic bones due to natural ligamentous changes that occur during pregnancy and can refer pain to the clitoral region. Another cause of postpartum clitoral pain may be due to tissue stresses that occur during a vaginal birth that can result in bruising, swelling, tears, or lacerations directly on or around the clitoris. While tears often occur near the bottom of the vaginal opening and at the perineum, they may extend upward toward the labia minora, urethra, or clitoris. Depending on the depth and extent of the tear, stitches may be used to promote complete tissue healing. As the body heals from any tear, scar tissue will form as part of the body's natural healing process.

Sometimes scars become tough and immobile, resulting in adherence, stiffness, and limited movement or retraction of the tissue. In this case, movement and massage around the labia minora, which connect directly around the clitoris to form the clitoral hood, can reduce clitoral pain. Additionally sitz baths, applying ice, avoiding direct stimulation of the affected area by refraining from masturbation and intercourse, avoiding abrasive materials when washing, wearing loose-fitting clothing, modifying some movements and positions, and initiating isometric exercises can all aid in comfort and time required for healing.

## Rectum

The rectum is the last several inches of the large intestine that stores feces in preparation for elimination. It's surrounded directly by the uterus in front and the sacrum in back and is supported by specific ligaments and pelvic floor muscles. Since the pelvic organs are positioned so closely to one another within the confined space of the pelvic cavity, the contents of any of the organs can affect function and mobility of the others around them.

Some common conditions that affect the rectum during pregnancy, birth, and the postpartum period include constipation, hemorrhoids, diarrhea, and bowel incontinence. During the postpartum period these symptoms can occur because of uterine contractions as the uterus begins to shrink after birth, and as a result of hormonal changes. Other issues with pelvic floor muscles can also contribute to these conditions. Pain medications can cause constipation, leading to elevated pressure in the rectum, causing hemorrhoids to develop.

Typically, changes affecting the bowels and GI system should begin to resolve within a few weeks following birth. If you experience constipation, movement and gentle exercise, dietary changes, taking specific supplements, and working with a pelvic physical therapist can all be effective in making lasting improvements. While common, taking stool softeners and laxatives as a long-term solution is not recommended as this could develop a dependency and lead to dehydration, mineral imbalance, and diarrhea. If you experience loose stool, evaluation by a trained pelvic physical therapist is recommended to help identify and address any pelvic floor or GI issues that may be contributing to your symptoms.

# Anatomy of the Hip Joint

## Bony Anatomy of the Hip Joint

The hip joint is the connection of the leg to the pelvis and is closely associated with the pelvic floor. The thigh bone (femur) is a long bone that connects to the lower leg (tibia) and knee (patella) at one end, and to the hip socket (acetabulum) of the pelvis at the other end. The femoral neck is a short segment of bone that connects the femoral shaft to the rounded ball of the femur, the femoral head. The femoral head fits within the concave surface of the acetabulum to create the hip joint (femoroacetabular joint) on each side of the pelvis.

You can easily locate your own hip joint in a standing position. Stand with your feet hip distance apart and arms straight at your sides. Use the webbing between your right thumb and index finger in a wide V position to locate the top rim of your pelvis, the iliac crest. Using moderate pressure from your flattened palm, slide down the outside of your thigh a few inches below the iliac crest. Rotate your right leg in and out and feel for

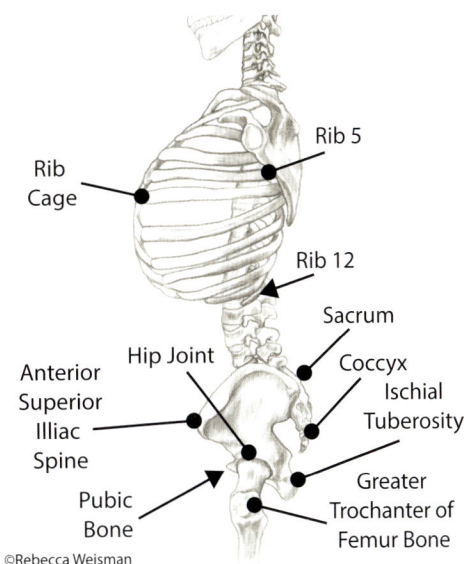

**FIGURE 1.16.** **Lateral view of the spine and pelvis**

a slightly raised area beneath your palm as your leg turns in. As you turn your leg out, notice that this raised area disappears. You have found your greater trochanter, a prominent ridge on the outside of the femur bone that is slightly forward and to the outside of your hip joint. Imagine a line from the greater trochanter slightly back and in toward the center of the body and you will be able to visualize the femoral neck and head coming in contact with the acetabulum. Compare the location of your greater trochanter on each side to estimate whether your hip joints are positioned in alignment with each other.

Since the head of the femur is larger than the hip socket is deep, a horseshoe-shaped cartilaginous tissue called the hip labrum lines and extends out from the acetabulum, deepening the socket and helping hold the femoral head in place in the center of the joint. The design of the ball-and-socket joint of the hip allows for many degrees of motion in multiple planes. Certain muscular, ligamentous, or tendinous variables can affect a person's range of motion, allowing for either more or less available movement. Range of motion can be influenced by exercise, strengthening, yoga, and other noninvasive techniques.

There are some limitations of movement at the hip joint that are in fact due to fixed or bony structural factors that will not change no matter how much stretching, mobilization, or manipulation a person undergoes, and therefore should not be forced. Femoral version, the angle of rotation of the femur bone, is one such factor. Its value is determined by measuring the angle of the neck of the femur in relation to the femoral condyles at the end of the bone near the knees, and on average it is between 10 and 20 degrees.[7] An angle greater than 20 degrees refers to anteversion and may present as a toed-in stance. An angle less than 10 degrees refers to retroversion and may present as a toed-out stance. These toed-in and toed-out presentations are natural compensatory patterns that bring the head of the femur into better contact with the acetabulum, which stabilizes the hip joint.

A person who presents with femoral anteversion will likely present with limited hip external rotation and should not force their hip into external rotation and abduction as this can result in injury to the hip labrum over time and with repetition. Likewise, a person with retroversion of their hip will have limitations with hip internal rotation. Getting screened by a physical therapist for these hip variations can help you become better educated and understand how to safely move, stretch, and strengthen without risking the integrity of the hip joint and its supportive structures.

Efforts to preserve the hip labrum should be considered specifically with birthing positions. The most common actions that the hip undergoes when birthing are flexion, abduction, and internal and external rotation. Extreme or forceful movements during labor and delivery can cause unnecessary injury to the hip joint, and specifically to the labrum. Though there are many effective positions a person can labor and birth in, lithotomy position (lying on your back with knees apart and legs supported in abduction and external rotation) is a very common position. Delivering in this position with outside forces applied to the hips in flexion, abduction, and rotation may affect the integrity of the hip labrum in the long term.[8]

While this may be a useful position for a person assisting with delivery of a baby, this is not necessarily the most optimal position for the person birthing a baby. Lying on your back blocks the sacrum from moving in a way that allows more space for the baby to pass through as it exits the pelvis. Alternative positions that allow for more sacral movement and potential space for the baby to pass through the pelvic outlet includes kneeling, squatting, lying on your side, or standing. Prior to delivery, consider and discuss alternative options for birthing positions, as it is important to avoid extremes that could compromise the labrum's integrity, particularly if medications that reduce sensation are used.

Hormonal changes can increase ligamentous laxity and contribute to less stability in the hip joint, placing elevated stress on the hip labrum. Developing stability in the surrounding hip musculature, learning alternative positions to labor and birth in, and learning which movements to avoid or modify during this process can help to preserve the labrum by lessening this stress. If you are postpartum and experiencing new hip pain, reflecting back and considering whether birthing positions are a factor in your pain can be helpful information in developing a plan of care with your pelvic floor physical therapist.

## Hip Rotators and Pelvic Nerves

The hip rotators are connected to the pelvic bones or sacrum at one end, and to the femur bone at the other. Fasciae, tendons, ligaments, and other connective tissues help connect and support the hip joint and allow for movement. A notable example of this influence can be seen by looking more closely at the obturator internus muscle. The obturator internus is an external rotator and abductor of the hip. Obturator internus attaches at one end to the inside of the bony pelvis on the internal surface of the obturator membrane and the bony boundaries of the obturator foramen, forming the side wall of the pelvis. It attaches at the other end to the greater trochanter, located on the outer femur. The obturator internus is separated from the true pelvic floor muscles by a thickened white fascial layer, the arcus tendineus levator ani, or ATLA, and arcus tendineus fascia pelvis, or ATFP. These fascial bands are points of attachment

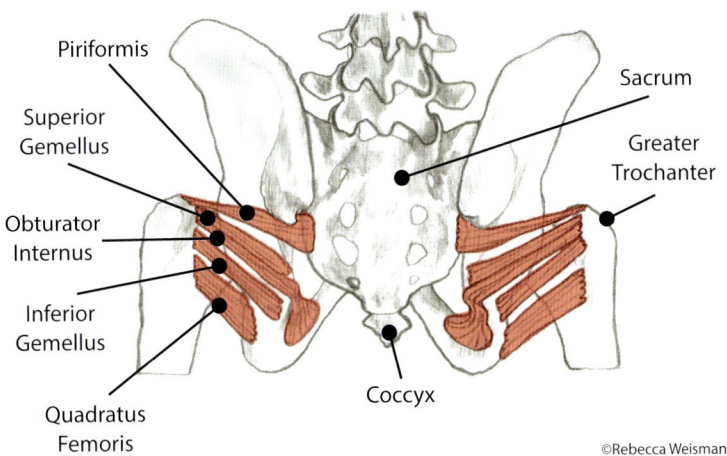

©Rebecca Weisman

**FIGURE 1.17.** Lateral hip rotators, posterior view

for the levator ani and endopelvic fascia, which is associated with support and function of the pelvic viscera.

Because of its anatomy, symptoms related to obturator internus involvement can be similar to those indicative of pelvic dysfunction, including reports of urinary frequency, groin or abdominal pain, sit bone or hip pain, and hamstring strain. For some with hamstring pain at the ischial attachments, obturator internus muscle tension should be ruled out as a cause or contributing factor to symptoms. If this muscle is found to be a factor, massage and self-release of the OI can be done by an individual externally where the muscle attaches at the obturator foramen of the pelvis. To find this area on your own, come to a seated position, place your hands underneath your buttocks, and locate the buttock bones. Curl your fingers around the inside of the bones and apply pressure to the muscles there, feeling for any tenderness or tightness. Tension or pain in this muscle can also be addressed internally with the help of a pelvic physical therapist and adaptive tools.

Another of the important lateral hip rotators is the piriformis muscle, the most superficial of the six short, deep rotator muscles of the hip. Piriformis is flat and, along with obturator internus, forms the posterior wall of the pelvis. It has attachments on the anterior surface of the sacrum, the posterior ilium, the sacrotuberous ligament, and the upper back surface of the greater trochanter of the femur bone. Piriformis externally rotates the femur, and it stabilizes the

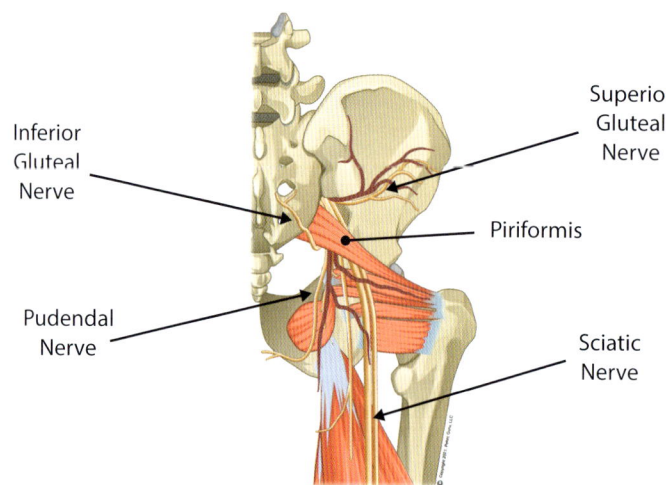

**FIGURE 1.18.** **Piriformis and pelvic nerves, posterior view**

head of the femur in the acetabulum. It also contributes to hip abduction when the hip is flexed.

Within the pelvic inlet and outlet are openings, the greater and lesser sciatic foramen, that are bounded by the sacrospinous and sacrotuberous ligaments, respectively. Many vessels and nerves pass through these openings to innervate muscles and tissues of the pelvis, hips, and lower extremities. Of note is the sciatic nerve (fig. 1.18). Because of their proximity to each other, if piriformis is tight or compressed, it could exert pressure on the sciatic nerve and cause pain, numbness, or even difficulty walking along the nerve distribution in the lower extremity. Piriformis muscle tension can increase during pregnancy, and after childbirth can contribute to imbalances in the pelvis. Poses such as Adho Mukha Swastikāsana, shown in Week 1 of the āsana practice section, chapter 2, may help reveal to you imbalances or places of tension.

Also important to note is the pudendal nerve, a peripheral nerve that arises from sacral nerve roots S2, S3, and S4. It sends and receives messages between your brain and your body regarding pelvic floor sensory and motor information. When this messaging system is intact, movement and sensation are undisturbed. However, whenever a nerve or tissue surrounding a nerve is compressed or irritated, problems can occur within this messaging system. Sensory or motor changes including pain, numbness, weakness, or bladder and bowel issues may occur. Some factors that could affect pudendal nerve function include a prolonged second stage of labor, use of delivery assistance tools, trauma to the area, prolonged sitting, tailbone injuries, chronic constipation, or surgery. Identifying issues driven by the pudendal nerve can be challenging, and if you suspect that it may be causing your symptoms, we encourage you to seek help from a medical provider or pelvic health specialist who is experienced with pudendal nerve conditions.

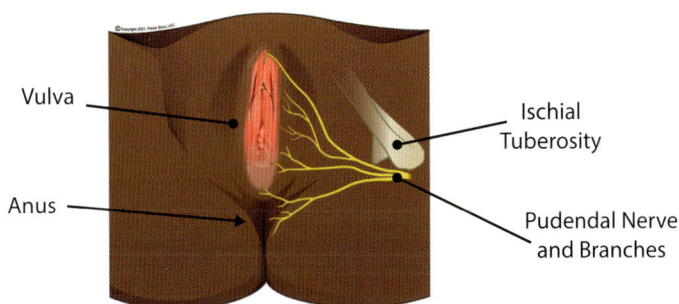

FIGURE 1.19. Pudendal nerve, inferior view

## Gluteal Muscles

Often referred to as buttock muscles, the gluteal muscles are located around the back outer portion of the pelvis and femur bone, and are close neighbors to the pelvic floor muscles. The glutes are a group of three distinct muscles: gluteus minimus, gluteus medius, and gluteus maximus, from deep to superficial. The glutes act on the hip joint and are mainly involved in extension (bringing the leg back) and abduction (bringing the leg out to the side, away from the midline). They also assist with other movements, including adduction (bringing the femur bone toward or across midline) and internal and external hip rotation (turning the thigh bone toward or away from midline, respectively). These muscles also play an important role in stabilizing the sacrum, walking, single leg standing, and negotiating stairs. Since these muscles are close neighbors to the pelvic floor muscles, it is important to consider how imbalances in one group of muscles may affect the other.

Gluteus minimus is the deepest of the three gluteal muscles and is an important pelvic stabilizer in bearing weight. It's a fan-shaped muscle that attaches to the femur bone at the greater trochanter and on the pelvis at the outer surface of the ilium bone. Along with gluteus medius, it stabilizes the pelvis during single limb support on the standing-leg side of the pelvis. This action prevents the pelvis from dropping on the opposite side, or the unweighted leg. Gluteus minimus also works to rotate the thigh bone inward, and when the femur is extended assists with external rotation.

Gluteus medius is also a fan-shaped muscle that is broader than and layered over the gluteus minimus. It also attaches to the greater trochanter of the femur bone and the ilium of the pelvis. Since it covers such a broad area, its muscle fibers contribute to different actions depending on the position of the thigh bone.

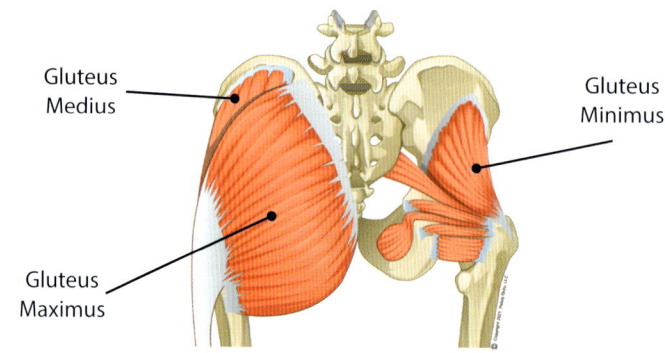

FIGURE 1.20.  **Gluteal muscles**

Gluteus medius's main action is hip abduction, moving the thigh bone away from the midline. This can be seen most easily during open-chain movements, when the leg is not bearing weight. An example of this is demonstrated in Ardha Chandrāsana as gluteus medius on the raised leg contracts to lift the raised leg.

Gluteus medius is also important as a hip stabilizer in a closed-chain position, when the leg is bearing weight. Using the same example of Ardha Chandrāsana, consider the action of the gluteus medius on the standing leg. Here the leg is fixed and the gluteus medius works to bring the pelvis closer to the femur, stabilizing the femur into the socket. Often yogic instructions to "compact" the hips in standing poses are actions that involve the gluteus medius. When both feet are weight-bearing, as in Tāḍāsana, gluteus minimus and gluteus medius could be considered the "core" of the hip as they provide support to stabilize the legs and pelvis.

Gluteus maximus is the largest and most superficial of the gluteal muscles. Gluteus maximus is an expansive and strong muscle that covers a large area of the pelvis, including the posterior pelvic bones, the gluteus medius, the upper hamstring muscles, and several layers of hip rotators. Its muscle fibers are oriented diagonally and laterally from the lateral and posterior surface of the sacrum and coccyx, the ilium, thoracolumbar fascia, and sacrotuberous ligament, and they attach to the lateral and posterior thigh bone and tensor fasciae latae. Actions of the gluteus maximus include hip extension, abduction, and external and internal rotation.

Since gluteus maximus attaches to the posterior (back) surface of the sacrum, and some of the deep pelvic floor muscles attach to the anterior (front) surface of the sacrum, these muscle groups counterbalance one another.[9] When the glutes are mobile and strong, they help to suspend the pelvic floor muscles and contribute to their trampoline-like quality. However, if the glutes are short or tight, they become weakened and cannot provide the movement or muscular counterbalance needed to suspend the pelvic floor. This can result in pelvic floor muscles becoming short, tight, and weak as the sacrum gets pulled closer to the pubic bone. Alternatively, if the glutes are overdeveloped, the sacrum can be pulled back, causing the pelvic muscles to overlengthen, becoming less mobile and weak.

Another factor to consider in the relationship between your glutes and pelvic floor muscles is unbalanced gluteal contraction on one side. Since the pelvic floor and gluteal muscles influence each other directly, gripping your glutes unequally could result in a similar imbalance of pelvic muscle tension. You may also observe connections between gluteal imbalances and other imbalances in your body, including in the legs, feet, and spine. This could be observed in lateral standing poses, as shown in Week 4 of the āsanas presented in chapter 2.

## Hamstrings

While the hamstring muscles are not part of the gluteal group of muscles, they play an important role assisting the glutes, hip rotators, and pelvic floor muscles. The hamstrings attach to the pelvis at the buttock bones on one end and cross the knee joint to attach on the back of the femur, the thigh bone, and the tibia and fibula, the lower leg bones. At the buttocks, portions of the hamstrings are overlapped by gluteus maximus. The hamstrings assist gluteus maximus with hip extension, and along with gluteus maximus provide counterbalance to other muscles acting on the pelvis, primarily the hip flexors. They work to stabilize the hip joint by maintaining some degree of hip extension so that the pelvis maintains a balanced position and doesn't just tip forward with the pull of the anterior chain of muscles. This is an important action for postpartum individuals, as it can be challenging to find a neutral position in the pelvis after pregnancy. The action of the hamstrings on the pelvis can be observed in poses such as Tāḍāsana or in Sālamba Sarvāṅgāsana, as shown in the Week 2 āsana practice section in chapter 2.

# Spine, Abdominals, and Core

## Bony Anatomy of the Spine

Another important neighbor to the pelvis is the spine. Range of motion in the spine affects, and is affected by, the pelvis and pelvic floor muscles. Overlapping fasciae and ligaments further support this interdependent relationship. The spinal column is located in the center of the body and spans vertically from the base of the head at one end to the sacrum at the other. It consists of individual stacked bones called vertebrae with discs in between for effective shock absorption, stress distribution, and movement. Ligaments situated along the entire length of the front and back of the spine connect and support the individual vertebrae and discs. The spine plays many important roles, allowing movement, providing protection for your spinal cord, and acting as a support system for the entire body, including the organs.

There are four specific regions of the spine where vertebrae vary in size, shape, design, and to some degree, function. From top to bottom they are the cervical,

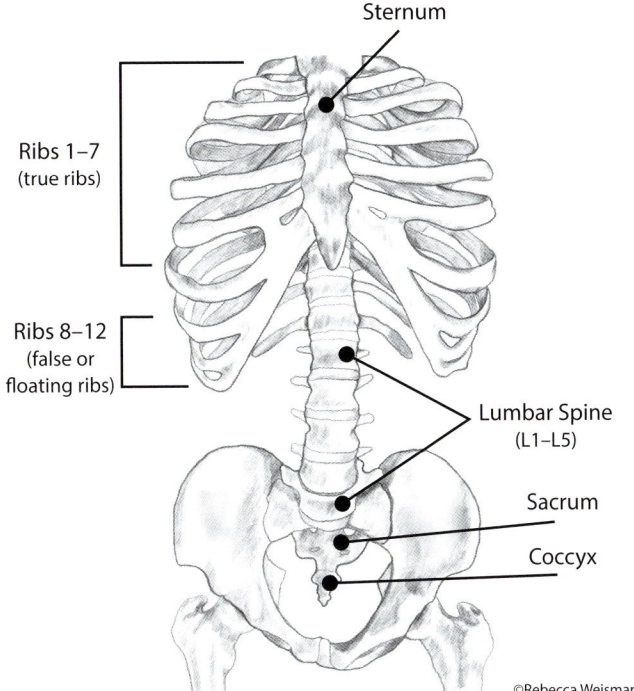

**FIGURE 1.21.**  **Anterior view of the spine**

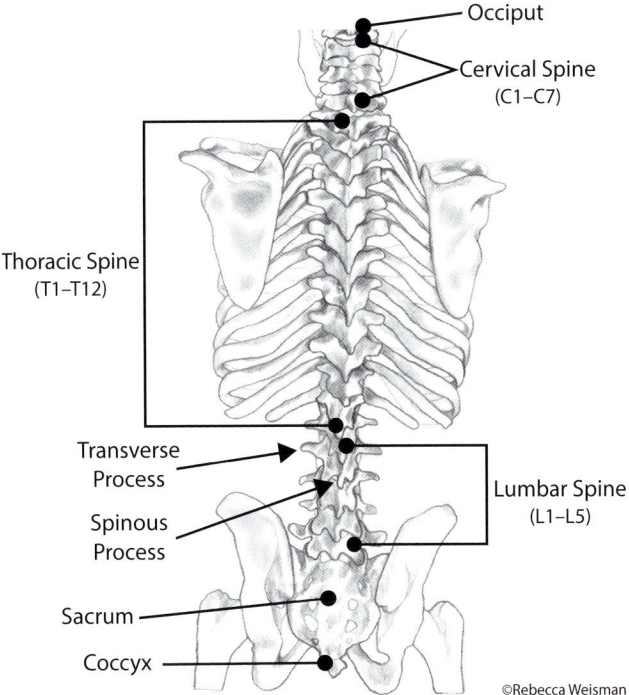

**FIGURE 1.22.**  **Posterior view of the spine**

thoracic, lumbar, and sacrococcygeal regions. Additionally, the spine has four natural curvatures that gradually alternate between concave and convex positions. The cervical spine has a concave curvature, and its primary movements are rotation, lateral flexion or side-bending, flexion, and extension. The thoracic region spans the largest area of the spine and is convex toward the upper and middle regions, beginning to transition toward concave in the lower region. This design allows primarily for rotation or twisting movements of the spine. The thoracic spine also connects with the ribs and influences breathing. The lumbar spine just below has concave curvature, and its primary movements are flexion and extension.

Finally, the sacrum has a convex shape. The movements that naturally occur at the sacrum are found where the 5th lumbar vertebra and top (called the base) of the sacrum meet, allowing a small degree of forward and backward movement. This is similar to flexion and extension, but in this part of the body, the movements are called nutation and counternutation, respectively. There is an even smaller amount of rotation between the sacrum and pelvic bones, and a tiny amount of side-bending on each side.[10] The spaces between the sacrum and pelvic bones on each side are the sacroiliac joints (SIJ). Held in place primarily by a network of ligamentous supports, the sacroiliac joints connect the spine to the pelvis and allow for transfer of weight from the lumbar spine to the lower extremities. If the support or position of the sacroiliac joint is interrupted or disturbed, as may occur with soft tissue injury, too much or too little mobility in the tissue, or typical changes that occur during pregnancy and delivery, you may experience sacroiliac joint instability or pain, or pelvic floor dysfunction.

Another common challenge for postpartum individuals is lower back pain, which may occur alongside sacroiliac joint symptoms. Lower back pain can be exacerbated by restricted movement in the thoracic spine. Breastfeeding and carrying babies also contributes to tightness in the upper back and can further stress the lumbar spine. These are just some examples of how the various parts of the spine and pelvis can influence one another. Understanding the movements and various structures of the spine may help you better understand the relationship between imbalances or symptoms in your spine and your pelvic floor.

Connected to the bottom of the sacrum is the coccyx, or tailbone, where a small degree of flexion and extension is possible at the sacrococcygeal joint. Like the other pelvic and spinal joints, it is reinforced in front and back by a ligamentous system. As noted previously, the coccyx plays an important role in pelvic floor function based on its location within the pelvis. The sacrococcygeal joint allows for movement of the coccyx during vaginal childbirth, and the coccyx can become displaced or even fractured. It is possible for the pelvis to remain in an open birthing pattern, in which the pelvic bones, sacrum, or coccyx shift position and do not automatically return to their pre-birth position.[11] Alternatively, the joint may settle into an imbalanced or less than optimum position during the postpartum period. These imbalances can affect the organization, support, function, and health of your pelvis. Taking time to learn about, visualize, and feel these structures in your own body can help guide you in your yoga practice and in determining whether to seek help from a pelvic floor physical therapist or other qualified professional.

## The Abdominal Container

When we work with new parents at any time following their birth experience, we often ask them to share what their goals are. "Getting my core back" is a response we hear over and over again. Before beginning this task, it is helpful to define what is meant by the term *core*. In the context of this book, the term refers to the coordination of a system of muscles that are found in your body between the respiratory diaphragm muscle, located within and around the perimeter of your rib cage, and the pelvic floor muscles. It also includes muscles in the front and back of the body, specifically the deepest layer of abdominals, the transverse abdominis, and deep spinal muscles called the multifidus. Together, these four groups of muscles create a physical container that encompasses the lower thoracic spine, the entirety of your lumbar spine, and the pelvis, and when they are working together, they act as an anticipatory system to prepare you for movement. Teaching these muscles to work together is a necessary first step in creating stability and efficiency of movement in the core. These deep muscles are surrounded by the internal and external obliques, rectus abdominis, erector spinae, and quadratus lumborum, which further reinforce the abdominal container.

From superficial to deep, the abdominal muscles are the rectus abdominis (RA), external oblique (EO), internal oblique (IO), and transverse abdominis (TA). The rectus abdominis muscle fibers are vertically oriented and occupy the midline of the anterior trunk with attachments at the pubic symphysis, pubic crest, pubic tubercle, xiphoid process of the sternum, and the costal cartilages of ribs 5 to 7.[12] Commonly thought of as the "abs" or "six-pack muscles," the rectus abdominis flexes or bends the trunk forward, assists with breathing, and helps compress or contain the abdominal organs. Through the center of the rectus abdominis is a long fibrous band called the linea alba, which stabilizes the anterior abdominal wall and separates the muscle into right and left sides.

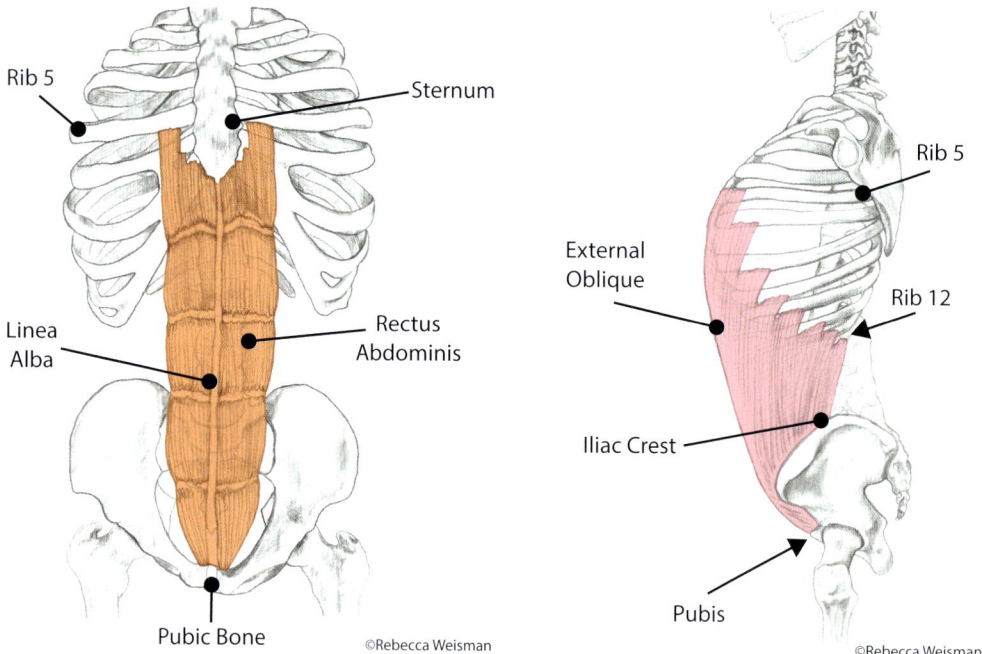

FIGURE 1.23. **Rectus abdominis.**

FIGURE 1.24. **External oblique**

During pregnancy, as the baby and uterus grow, some people develop a separation of the linea alba. This is called a diastasis recti abdominis and is discussed in more detail in chapter 3.

The external obliques are the most superficial of the lateral group of abdominal muscles. With diagonally oriented muscle fibers, angled down and in laterally to medially, the external obliques cover the internal obliques and the front of the lower ribs and intercostal muscles, making up part of the lateral abdominal wall. Along with the internal obliques, they contribute to trunk rotation to the opposite side and lateral flexion of the trunk to the same side. They also assist the rectus abdominis and the internal obliques in trunk flexion or forward bending, which elevates intra-abdominal pressure and supports physiologic processes such as forced exhalation, defecation, urination, and labor.[13]

The next layer of abdominals deep to the external obliques are the internal oblique muscles, with diagonally oriented fibers directed down and out from medial to lateral attachments. Similarly to the external obliques, the internal obliques contribute to trunk flexion or forward bending and visceral compression when both sides are activated at the same time. When one side is activated at a time, they support trunk side-bending and rotation. The internal obliques also maintain normal abdominal tension and forceful exhalation.

The transverse abdominis (TA) muscle is the deepest of the four layers of abdominal muscle, and along with the rectus abdominis makes up the front and sides of the abdominal wall. The transverse abdominis connects to the lower six ribs, the front of the iliac crest and pubis, and the thoracolumbar fascia in the back.[14] The muscle fibers are oriented horizontally, or transversely, and are situated perpendicular to the linea alba. Appreciate how the transverse abdominis creates a container-like wrapping from the front toward the back, providing stability at a deep layer. Along with the other abdominal muscles, transverse abdominis is responsible for maintaining normal abdominal tension and balances intra-abdominal pressure. Engagement of these muscles supports exhalation, helps contain abdominal viscera, and assists in stabilizing the spine and pelvis in preparation for movement. Also appreciate how each layer of the abdominals overlaps, with muscle fibers oriented in various directions to provide reinforcement of this container.

While technically the iliopsoas is not part of the core group of muscles, it provides structural and postural support for the curves of the spine and forms the back wall of the abdominal container, where it supports the abdominal organs. The iliopsoas is a group of three muscles: psoas major, psoas minor, and iliacus. Together, psoas major and minor attach and span the distance between the twelfth thoracic vertebra (T12) and the fifth lumbar vertebra (L5) on each side of

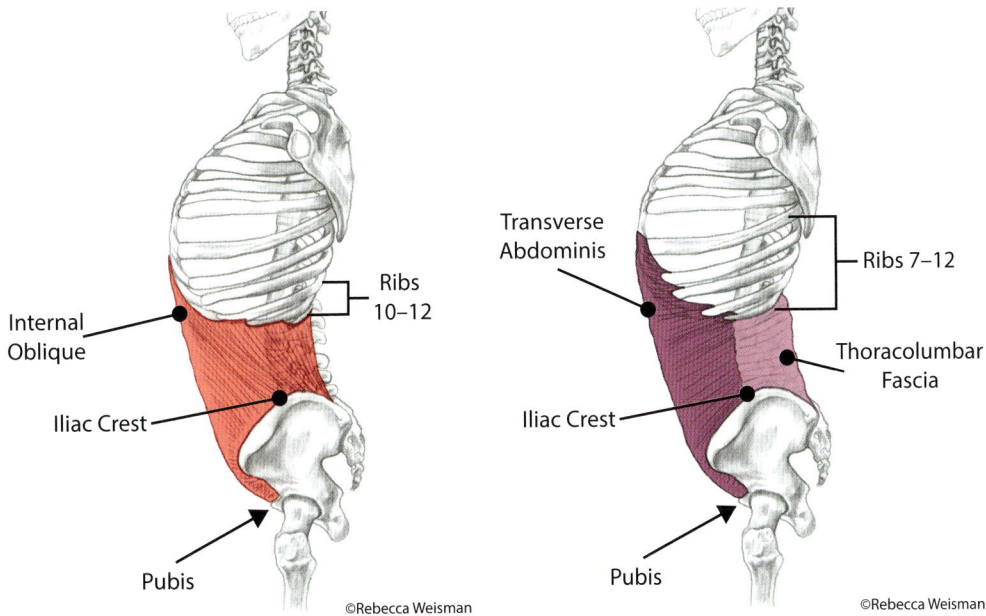

Internal
Oblique

Ribs
10–12

Iliac Crest

Pubis

©Rebecca Weisman

**FIGURE 1.25. Internal oblique**

Transverse
Abdominis

Ribs 7–12

Thoracolumbar
Fascia

Iliac Crest

Pubis

©Rebecca Weisman

**FIGURE 1.26. Transverse abdominis**

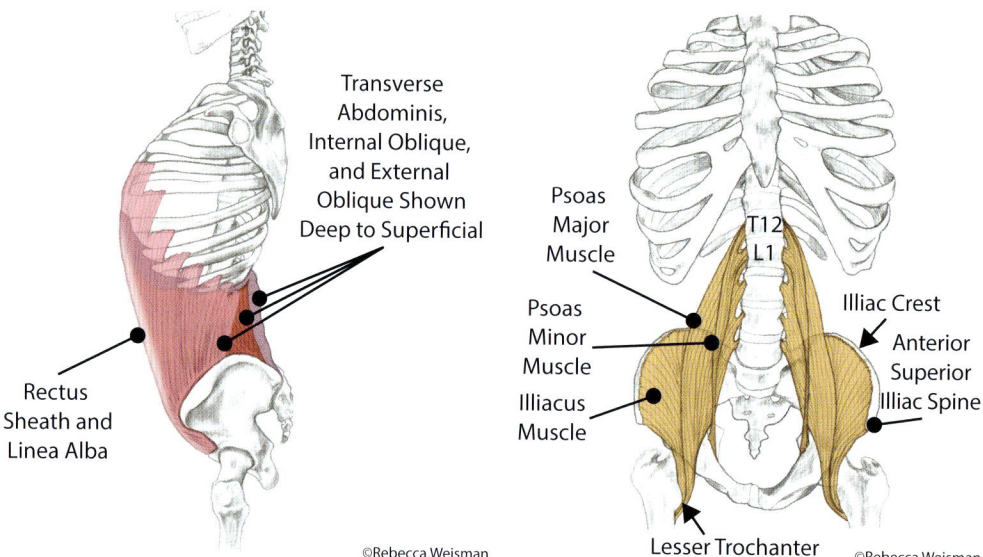

Transverse Abdominis, Internal Oblique, and External Oblique Shown Deep to Superficial

Rectus Sheath and Linea Alba

©Rebecca Weisman

Psoas Major Muscle

Psoas Minor Muscle

Illiacus Muscle

T12 L1

Illiac Crest

Anterior Superior Illiac Spine

Lesser Trochanter

©Rebecca Weisman

**FIGURE 1.27. All four layers of the lateral abdominal muscles**

**FIGURE 1.28. Iliopsoas**

the spine. Here these muscles join with the iliacus, a fan-shaped muscle on the front surface of the ilium, cross over the front of the pelvis, and attach to the inner upper surface of the femur. The iliopsoas is a major hip flexor and contributes to hip external rotation. It is the only muscle that connects your spine directly to your leg and therefore plays a huge role in posture, standing, and walking.

Following the processes of pregnancy and birth, imbalances in the pelvis and spine are commonly experienced, resulting in a lack of stability and support. For many people the iliopsoas can become short and tight during pregnancy as the body adapts to changes in the size, shape, weight, and position of the uterus. For some people, the iliopsoas muscle compensates for the lack of stability in the pelvic joints, lack of control or engagement in the pelvic floor, or lack of support from the core muscles. Following pregnancy, stretching and strengthening these muscles in elongated positions can be helpful, as explored in chapter 2.

## Diaphragms, Breathing, and Pressures

Throughout your body are spaces or cavities that house your organs and vital structures. The pelvic cavity contains the corresponding organs, the abdominal cavity holds all of your abdominal viscera, and your thoracic cavity is home to the heart and lungs. Each of these cavities and their contents are separated from one another by diaphragms. The word *diaphragm* refers to a separation or a divide constructed mostly of fascial and muscular bands of tissue that separate cavities in your body. We also use the word diaphragm to refer to the respiratory diaphragm muscle, which is a discrete muscle in the body that also acts as a partition. There are two main diaphragms that influence pelvic health: the pelvic diaphragm and the thoracic or respiratory diaphragm. Your pelvic diaphragm separates the abdominal cavity from the pelvic bowl and is demarcated by a thin layer of tissue, and the thoracic diaphragm separates the abdominal cavity from the thoracic cavity above and is demarcated by the respiratory diaphragm muscle.

The throat acts like a third diaphragm, and there can be interplay between the vocal folds and the lower diaphragms with respect to pelvic health. The vocal folds move more laterally than the other two diaphragms, widening and

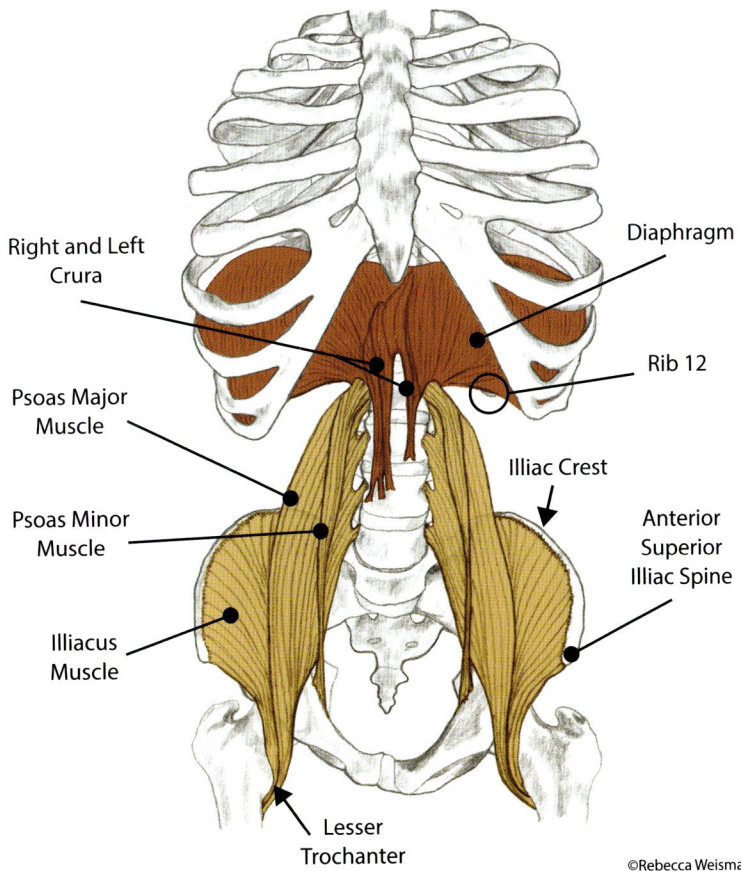

©Rebecca Weisman

**FIGURE 1.29.** **Respiratory diaphragm showing overlap with the iliopsoas muscle, anterior view**

narrowing to either open or seal the trachea, or windpipe. Further, the vocal folds vibrate, alternately holding and releasing air, which can aid in overall relaxation.[15] It is because of this connection that low-pitched sounds are often encouraged to assist with birthing a baby. Making steady, low-pitched sounds may be helpful for reeducating pelvic muscle and nervous system connections in people who experience tension in their pelvic muscles. With high vocal cord vocalization, on the other hand, the jaw and pelvic floor muscles receive signals from the nervous system for muscles to contract, creating muscle tension. This may be useful for someone with reduced muscle tension to refine and reeducate the connection between the nervous system and muscular system in this way.

In addition to muscle length, alignment plays a significant role in the efficiency and function of the diaphragms. From a standing position, notice that your pelvic and thoracic diaphragms as well as your vocal folds are relatively stacked in the body, one above the other. If the muscles and surrounding tissues of the diaphragms are mobile and can move through their full range of motion, contracting and releasing completely, smooth and efficient exchange of pressures within and between your cavities can occur. However, if the muscle and tissue movement is restricted or the diaphragms are misaligned, you may feel resistance or restriction in your pelvis, trunk, neck, or elsewhere in the body, and restriction in breathing. In this way, alignment and posture can influence your efficiency of breathing. While the diaphragms create some physical separation, it's important that they are able to communicate and respond to one another in order to manage pressures throughout each of their spaces effectively.

## The Respiratory Diaphragm

The respiratory diaphragm is one of the main muscles of respiration. It is a dome-shaped muscle located in the trunk that acts as a separation between the abdominal and thoracic cavities and their respective organs, the heart and lungs above and the abdominal contents below. It attaches to its own central tendon at the top of the dome, the xiphoid process of the sternum and the costal cartilage of ribs 7 to 12 in front, to the 11th and 12th ribs laterally, to vertebrae L1 to L3 in the back, and to the anterior longitudinal ligament along the front of the spine, where it overlaps with tendinous attachments of the psoas major muscle.[16] Take a moment to appreciate this overlap and connections between possible tension at the iliopsoas, restricted breathing, and the sympathetic nervous system or a fight-flight-freeze response, discussed in more detail below.

During inspiration, your respiratory diaphragm muscle contracts, and the shape of the thoracic cavity changes as the muscle moves down and broadens toward the abdomen and its organic contents. This increases the volume of the thoracic cavity and reduces pressure within the lungs, allowing air to flow in. At the same time, a pressure change occurs in the abdominal cavity, increasing intra-abdominal pressure. Visually, the chest inflates, the ribs expand, and the abdomen rises.

During expiration, the respiratory diaphragm relaxes. It moves up and in toward the center, returning to its dome-like shape. This reduces thoracic volume and elevates pressure within the lungs, pushing air out, and intra-abdominal pressure decreases. Visually the chest recedes, and the abdomen descends.

## Breathing and the Pelvic Floor Muscles

While, technically speaking, the pelvic floor muscles are not synonymous with the pelvic diaphragm, they are often referred to as a diaphragm because how they move plays an important role in balancing pressures inside the body. The pelvic muscles should align and move in synchrony with the respiratory diaphragm. During inspiration, the pelvic floor muscles relax and should broaden and descend through their full range of motion. During expiration, they contract, lifting and narrowing. These movements aid the pressure changes throughout your pelvic, abdominal, and thoracic cavities, and provide balance and support in a constantly changing environment.

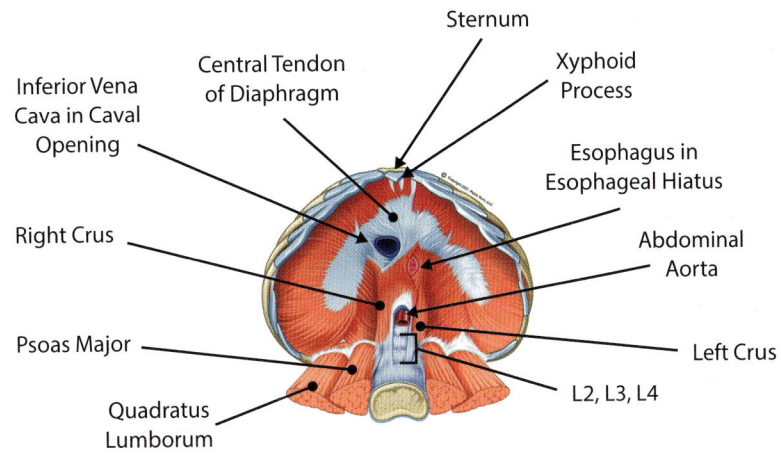

**FIGURE 1.30. Respiratory diaphragm, inferior view**

It is important to understand and learn this synchronization of movement between the respiratory diaphragm and the pelvic floor muscles, the practice of which we cover in more depth in chapter 2. In addition, consider the role your breath plays in connection to your nervous system. Your breath is regulated by your autonomic nervous system, the part of your nervous system that controls involuntary physiologic processes, including heart rate, blood pressure, digestion, sexual arousal, and respiration. Slow, steady, extended exhalation stimulates the vagus nerve and activates your parasympathetic nervous system, also known as your rest and digest system.[17] In contrast, shallow, quick breathing stimulates your sympathetic nervous system, commonly referred to as your flight, fight, or freeze system.

While both these systems are important and necessary for survival, they are not always in a perfect state of balance. Daily experiences in life may create changes in the balance of these systems. However,

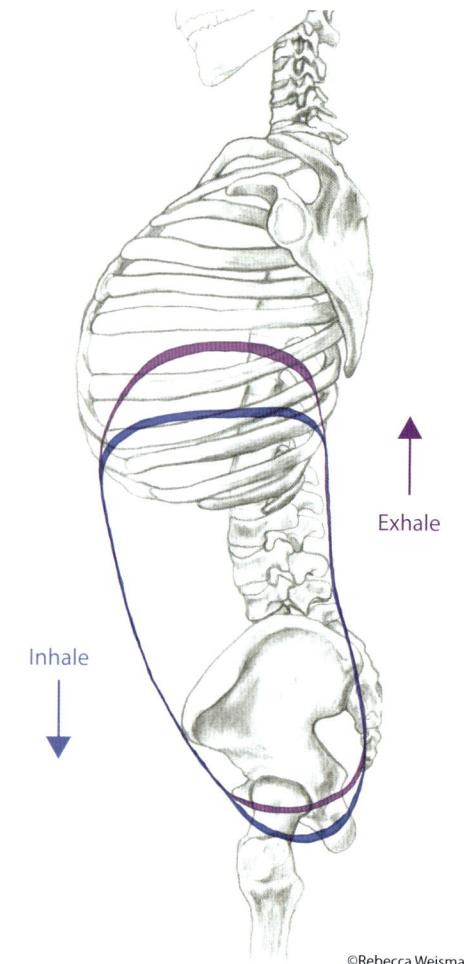

©Rebecca Weisman

**FIGURE 1.31.** **Respiration showing the coordinated direction of movements of the respiratory diaphragm and the pelvic floor muscles**

once an experience, thought, emotion, or feeling has passed, these systems should return to their baseline state in order to continue to respond in a reliable and helpful manner for optimal health. While this may sound simple enough, in reality we all encounter obstacles to establishing balance in our nervous system. This is especially true during the postpartum period, in which the body, including the nervous system, is recovering from a major event, and in which you are not always getting adequate rest, nutrition, and relaxation. Working with your breath daily is an easy place to start to balance your nervous system, and to begin to create balance in intra-abdominal and pelvic pressures. Below are some simple exercises to begin observing your breath.

Take note if breathing into your chest and abdomen feels unfamiliar or whether the movement suggested is opposite of what you expect. For many people, the movement and coordination of breath has become mixed up over the years for any number of reasons. As a result, you may use a reverse or paradoxical breathing pattern where, for example, the abdomen and abdominal pressures draw in and up when you inhale and move down and out when you exhale. As we'll see later in this book, this reverse breathing pattern creates imbalanced pressures in the cavities of the body and restricts the movement necessary to maintain a dynamic core system. Additionally, if you noticed your abdomen inflating much more than your chest, you may be unintentionally creating too much downward pressure with your inhalation, which can have negative effects on the abdominal and pelvic organs. Repeat these exercises daily until you feel more balance in these areas. For more specific breath instruction, see Week 1 in chapter 2.

## EXERCISE 1. OBSERVING YOUR BREATH AT REST

Lie down in a comfortable position with one hand on your abdomen and one hand on your chest. Begin to follow your breath without directing it.

Notice the movement, speed, and depth of your own breath. Where do you feel or notice movement or stillness?

When you breathe in, what direction does your abdomen move? Your chest?

What happens when you breathe out?

## EXERCISE 2. COORDINATING MOVEMENT OF YOUR ABDOMEN AND CHEST

You should notice a subtle rise in your abdomen and your chest as you breathe in, and a subtle fall as you breathe out. Can you feel these movements? Continue working to improve coordination.

# Conclusion

While there are a lot of different elements to your anatomy, understanding the different parts and being able to conceptualize, visualize, and feel them all together will help you deepen your relationship and connection to how these systems present and perform in your own body. There is a lot of information here that can be useful to refer back to, and we encourage you to reread pertinent sections as you practice and as you explore your own pelvis. Sometimes you may feel something different from what is described, and that is also OK! Try to be curious about your experience and recognize that all bodies are different, and each person's individual situation will be different. It is not unusual to feel confused about your pelvic floor, and we hope that the information here will help you home in on and give language to any specific parts of the body where you may be experiencing pain or symptoms. Additionally, we encourage you to use this information as a launching point to seek further guidance from professionals.

# SEQUENCES *of* ĀSANAS *for* PRACTICE

## Introduction to Āsana and Prāṇāyāma

The poses in this book are based on the principles of Iyengar Yoga. The sequences have been intentionally kept simple, straightforward, and manageable even for beginners or those with limited time. Some props will be helpful, such as three blankets, two blocks, a belt, a bolster, and a chair. Efforts have been made to keep the prop setups to a minimum to help with accessing and experiencing the poses more easily. Oftentimes, regular household items can be used, like firm pillows or cushions. For those with more experience, or those with specific symptoms that affect the hip or back, extra props may be used to make a pose therapeutic and most beneficial. Any pose that causes pain should be avoided, and it is recommended that you work with this manual under the supervision of your local Certified Iyengar Yoga Teacher to optimize the therapeutic benefits of the poses.

The poses here are broken into seven weeks of sequences, but you will likely need to proceed much more slowly than that, taking several weeks to work on each sequence. In other words, we are not referring to the number of weeks postpartum but to a progression of learning that you might undertake when you are ready. Each sequence is progressive, meaning it builds on the learning in the previous sequence, and care should be taken not to rush.

We recommend that you begin with the Week 1 poses and spend several weeks acquainting yourself with these poses and the specific *actions* within the poses before moving on. Furthermore, those who are newly postpartum may find they need to go through the sequences more slowly to allow more time for healing. Each sequence gives more specific guidance about timing and how long to wait postpartum before attempting the āsanas in each section. Some sequences may bring substantial relief, or you may find a "golden pose" that relieves pain or helps build awareness. Practitioners may want to spend time focusing on those poses and sequences that are most beneficial. Remember, this is *your* pelvic floor journey, and we encourage you to work at your own pace.

# Week 1

# CONNECTION THROUGH BREATH *and* RESTORATIVE ĀSANAS

The first step on embarking on your pelvic floor journey is to reconnect with this area of the body. For many people it is hard to sense or visualize, feels taboo or disconnected, or is simply outside their field of perception. While our anatomy sections help you to understand intellectually the various bones, joints, muscles, ligaments, and organs associated with the pelvis, these diagrams are not enough to allow you to truly *feel* what is happening inside your body. One of the main principles of yoga is that our perceptive awareness and our physical, material body are not separate, but linked in important ways. This link between the physiological body, breath, and our awareness is important to nurture if we want to connect with and eventually heal our pelvic floor.

In this chapter we focus on how to use the breath and restorative poses to begin to sense and map out your pelvic floor. We call this process *getting to know your pelvic floor landscape*. Just as you might take time getting to know the hills, valleys, and roadways of a new terrain, it will take some time for you to become acquainted with your pelvic floor. With patience and practice, this sequence will guide you in learning to synchronize your breath with your pelvic floor movements, address tension in the pelvic floor, and develop deepened awareness and comfort.

Restorative āsanas are extremely important for people recovering from childbirth as well as for anyone learning the initial relaxation and breathing that is key to understanding pelvic floor health. Contrary to common belief, pelvic health should not automatically start with strengthening. While strengthening has its place (see Week 3), many people struggle with symptoms related to high tension in the pelvic floor muscles. This can be due to traumatic birth, previous injuries and chronic pain, compensation for weak muscles elsewhere, stress, or structural imbalances. Elevated tension in the pelvic floor muscles can contribute to a variety of pelvic symptoms including general pain, pain during intercourse, difficulty with elimination, and pain in the hip, sacrum, or lower back.

In these cases, the first step in bringing balance to the pelvic floor is to release tension. Even those who have weakness will benefit from learning to relax and release the pelvic floor muscles, as this is necessary to regain or maintain the full range of motion in these muscle fibers.

Further, those who have recently given birth often do not get the adequate rest and nourishment needed for optimum healing. Sleep deprivation and the tolls of caring for a newborn can create a heightened urgency or stress in the nervous system, which can contribute to tension in the pelvic floor. Some people find that their yoga practice is the only time they feel truly relaxed and rested. Even just a few minutes each day of focused relaxation can aid in the healing process.

But you may be asking, "How do I know whether my muscles have too much or too little tension?" While this sequence is designed to help you gain aware-ness of your pelvic floor "landscape," there are a few other tools that may be ben-eficial. You may have access to a pelvic floor physical therapist who can do an internal assessment and help you determine any areas that may be tight, painful, or weak. You can also do your own internal assessment. Many people may feel timid or shy to do their own internal assessment, but it can be an empower-ing and eye-opening experience, and a tool that you can continue to use as you progress on your pelvic floor journey. See "Pelvic Floor Muscles" in chapter 1 for specific guidance about how to do an internal assessment on your own.

Even with all these tools, you may still feel in the dark about the nature of your pelvic floor. That's OK! Many students we've taught, even advanced prac-titioners, say they don't really know where it is or what to feel for. We encourage you just to make a start and trust that awareness will build with practice. The sequence of āsanas in this section and the accompanying instructions will help you learn how to relax the pelvic floor and abdomen and use the breath in con-junction with the movements of the pelvic and respiratory diaphragms. Post-partum people can begin with this sequence a few weeks after childbirth, once the bleeding has diminished, except for Viparīta Karaṇī, which should only be practiced after bleeding has completely stopped. Those who have delivered via cesarean should wait longer, six to eight weeks or with the approval of your medical provider, and then should proceed with caution. If perineal tearing has occurred, wait until the tear has completely healed, and then you may need to proceed cautiously in any pose that spreads the legs and groins laterally.

Postpartum individuals should focus on **the poses that feel best,** even if it is only one or two poses to begin with, rather than striving to complete the full sequence. Do not do any poses that create pain or that you do not feel ready for. This sequence can also be used during menstruation (except for Viparīta

Karaṇī). As with all of our sequences, consult your local Certified Iyengar Yoga Teacher if questions arise.

## Sequence of Āsanas: Week 1

### 1. ESTABLISHING YOUR BREATH

Lie down on the floor with a folded blanket under your head and your knees bent with the soles of your feet on the floor.. You can put a belt around your outer knees, hips width apart, and allow your knees to release away from each other, resting against the belt. Slow your breath, breathing evenly through the nose. Soften your eyes, your face and throat, tongue, teeth, chest, and abdomen. Observe the movements of your lower ribs and diaphragm. If it's helpful, you can place your hands on your lower ribs. Notice as you breathe in that the lower ribs expand outward, and the respiratory diaphragm moves slightly down toward the pelvis; as you exhale, the lower ribs narrow, and the diaphragm moves up toward the chest, away from the pelvis. Keep the belly soft and watch that you are not pushing your breath downward into the belly, but rather draw it slowly out to the sides. Repeat several cycles of breath this way.

Now bring your attention to your pelvic floor. What do you notice? Take several breaths and observe any movements or sensations in the pelvis. Visualize or feel your pelvic floor muscles moving with the same rhythm as your respiratory diaphragm and ribs. As you inhale, relax and broaden the pelvic floor muscles, and as you exhale, feel them gather in and slightly up. Keep your focus on the inhalation more than the exhalation, consciously releasing, spreading, and relaxing the pelvic floor muscles with the in-breath. Repeat several breaths like this.

At first, you may need to visualize the movements of the pelvic floor. If you get lost or confused, return to placing your hands on your ribs and feel or visualize

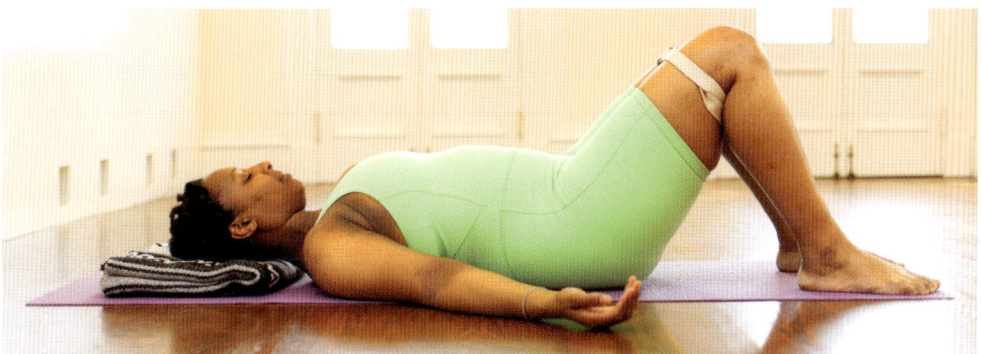

FIGURE 2.1. **Establishing your breath**

the movement of the respiratory diaphragm. The movement of the pelvic diaphragm should mirror the movement of the respiratory diaphragm. Observe:

Can you feel the respiratory diaphragm moving with the breath?

Can you feel the movements of the pelvic floor moving with your breath?

Can you synchronize your breath with your pelvic floor movement?

### 2. Supta Baddha Koṇāsana (Supine Bound Angle Pose)

Position the bolster lengthwise on the mat, and sit on the floor with the soles of the feet together, a few inches away from the edge of the bolster. Make a large loop of your belt and place it around the waist, over the root of the thighs, and slip it around the outer edges of your feet. Buckle the belt, pulling the feet in close to the groin. Support each thigh with a rolled blanket under the thigh and shin. Keeping the chest lifted, lie back over the bolster. Support the head and neck with a folded blanket. Lift the buttocks slightly and bring the tailbone toward the heels and the pubis toward the navel. Roll the outer upper arms down toward the floor and lengthen the shoulder blades down the back to open the chest. Rest with the palms up (figs. 2.2 and 2.3). Soften the abdomen and groins. Smooth out and soften the breath and make it even and rhythmic. Soften and gently spread the pelvic floor muscles on the inhalation, and on the exhalation feel a slight lift and return of those muscles, but don't contract. The pelvic floor muscles should move with the rhythm of the respiratory diaphragm. Observe any unevenness in the spreading of the pelvic floor muscles and relax any areas that are gripping, giving more attention to the spreading and relaxing effect on the inhalation. Stay for three to five minutes.

You should feel comfortable and supported in this āsana. If the groins are not soft, add more blankets under the thighs for more support. If the tailbone is not moving in, loosen the belt and move the feet slightly away from the groins, or support the thighs higher with additional blankets. If the abdomen is puffing or the pubis is dropping toward the floor, shift the bolster another inch or two away from the buttocks and move the tailbone in again. Also note, people who are newly postpartum should support the outer thighs with extra blankets so the spreading action of the hips and pelvis is lessened, gradually reducing the height of the blankets over several weeks.

### VARIATIONS

TWO-BELT VARIATION: If a second belt is available, belt each shin to the thigh independently, placing the belt around the root of the thigh and the

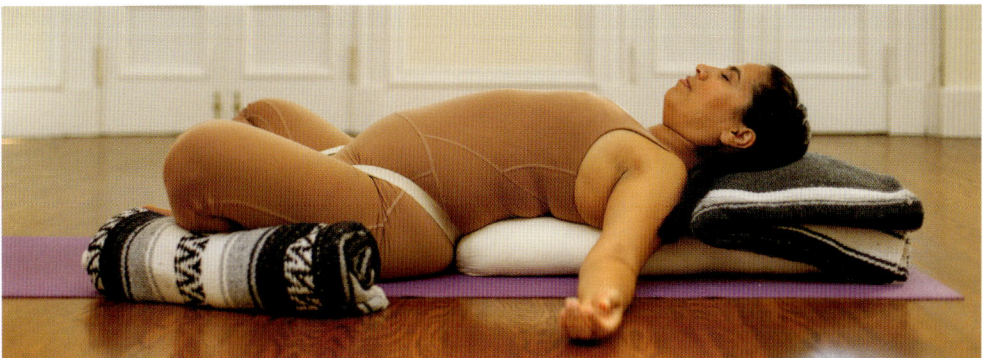

FIGURE 2.2. **Supta Baddha Koṇāsana**

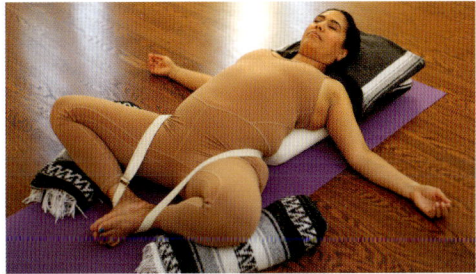

FIGURE 2.3. **Lengthwise bolster with a single belt**

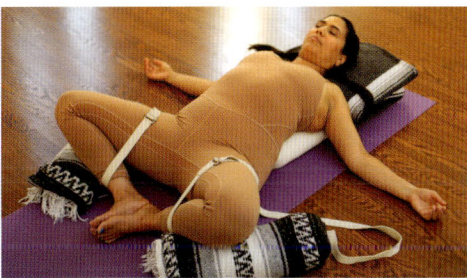

FIGURE 2.4. **Lengthwise bolster with two belts**

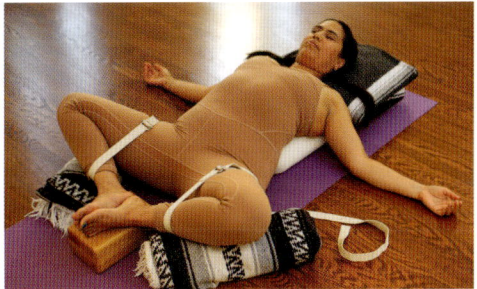

FIGURE 2.5. **Lengthwise bolster, two belts, feet on a block**

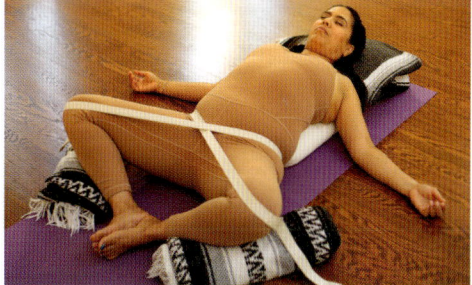

FIGURE 2.6. **Lengthwise bolster with crossed belts**

bottom of the shin bone, and tighten the belt with the buckle facing toward you (fig. 2.4). This variation gives superior spreading to the abdomen and lower back and may allow you to better adjust the tailbone toward the heels.

BACKACHE: Turn the bolster transverse and place it under the upper thoracic spine, adding a narrow-folded blanket on top for more height. Support the head on a block (medium or high height) or use a couple of thickly folded blankets placed behind the bolster (see the setup for Supta Vīrāsana in fig. 2.11). Some postpartum people may find it helpful to practice with the spine flat on the floor, with rolled blankets under the thighs and shins.

PELVIC OR HIP INSTABILITY: Use two belts, each one looped from the hip bone of one side of the pelvis to the knee of the opposite leg (fig. 2.6). This creates a more compacting action of the femur bone into the hip socket, and it can help ease some sacroiliac pain.

### 3. Supta Vīrāsana (Supine Hero's Pose)

Using the same bolster setup as in Supta Baddha Koṇāsana, sit a few inches in front of the bolster, with your buttocks between your heels, knees together, and toes pointing straight back. Place a belt around your thighs and shins just above the knees. Press your palms down to lift your chest and simultaneously move the tailbone and buttocks toward the knees as you lie back over the bolster (figs. 2.7 and 2.8). The sacrum should shift to be more parallel to the floor. Adjust your shoulder blades down your back and keep your chest open and spreading. For an intensified opening in the chest, stretch the arms overhead with the palms facing up for twenty to thirty seconds, and then release the arms back down by your sides.

Alternately, cross your forearms overhead, hold your elbows, and rest there for a short while, alternating your grip of the forearms or elbows (see figs. 2.10 and 2.13). Like in Supta Baddha Koṇāsana, even out your breathing. Soften and gently spread the pelvic floor muscles on the inhalation, and on the exhalation, feel a slight lift and return of those muscles, but don't contract. Observe any unevenness in the spreading of the pelvic floor muscles and relax any areas that are gripped, giving more attention to the spreading and relaxing effect on the inhalation. Stay for three to five minutes.

### VARIATIONS

TIGHT THIGHS OR KNEE PAIN: Sit on a flat block and support the spine higher by adding two narrow folded blankets on top of the bolster. Alternately, stack two bolsters, one atop the other, staggering them so the top bolster is farther back (figs. 2.9 and 2.10). Place a block under the far end of the top bolster to keep it in place. Sit on the edge of the bottom bolster and lie back.

BACKACHE: Turn the bolster transversely and place it under the upper thoracic spine (figs. 2.11 and 2.12). Support your head on a block (medium or high height) or use a couple of thickly folded blankets behind the bolster. If

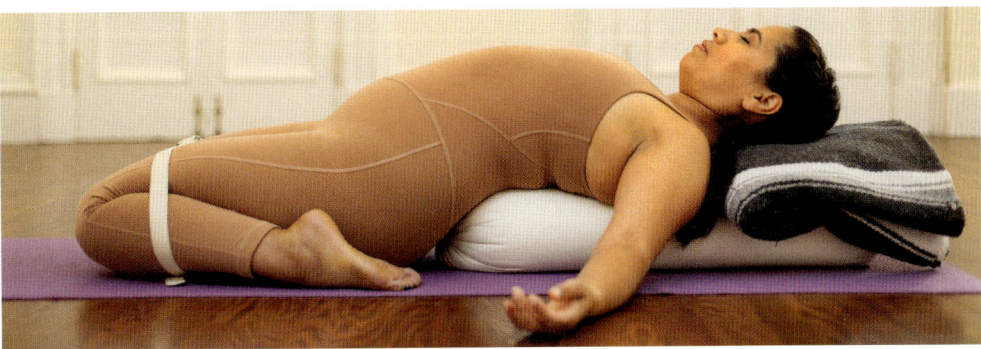

FIGURE 2.7. Supta Vīrāsana

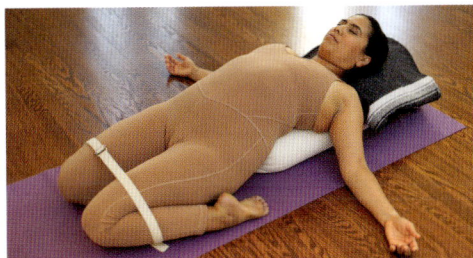

FIGURE 2.8. Lengthwise bolster

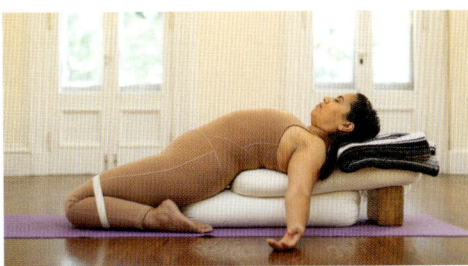

FIGURE 2.9. Additional height under the buttocks and torso

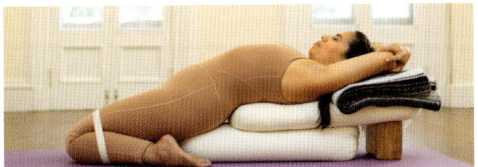

FIGURE 2.10. Additional height with arms overhead

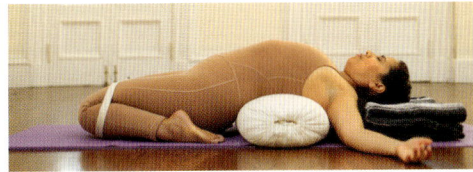

FIGURE 2.11. Transverse bolster

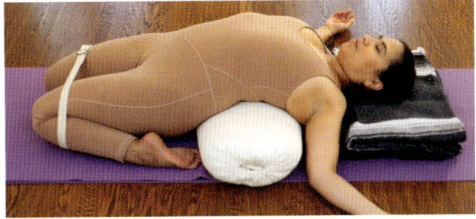

FIGURE 2.12. Transverse bolster (alternate view)

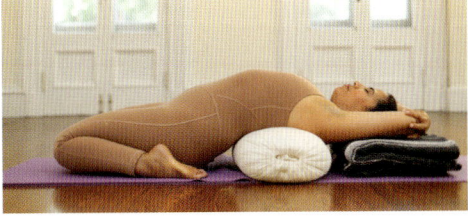

FIGURE 2.13. Transverse bolster with arms overhead

height is needed under the buttocks, place a block under the buttocks and add one or two narrow folded blankets to the bolster to increase the height under the chest. Additional height may be used for the head.

## 4. SUPTA SWASTIKĀSANA (SUPINE CROSSED LEGS)

Use the same setup as in the previous supine poses. Sit with your legs crossed at the center of your shin bones, feet directly under the knees. Lift the chest and bring the buttocks away from the lumbar spine as you lie back over the bolster (fig. 2.14). Spread your chest by rolling the upper outer arms down toward the floor, and move the shoulder blades down your back. Soften your breath and gently allow the pelvic floor muscles to spread. Observe the movements of the inhalation and exhalation in conjunction with the pelvic floor, again bringing more focus to spreading the pelvis on the inhalation. Stay for three to five minutes.

This pose should be comfortable and restful. If the groins don't feel relaxed, add a folded blanket between your foot and knee on each side. Two crossed belts can be used for more pelvic support and stability, as in the Supta Baddha Koṇāsana variation (fig. 2.6). Alternatively, if you only have one belt, belt one knee to the foot of the opposite leg that is supporting it, then twist the belt into a figure eight and belt the other knee and foot.

**Effects:** *These three supine poses help to gently soften the pelvic floor muscles, release the abdomen, and open the chest, allowing for more breath to reach these areas. You may feel more of a connection with the pelvic floor movements. These poses are also quieting for the mind and nervous system, and they help relieve fatigue.*

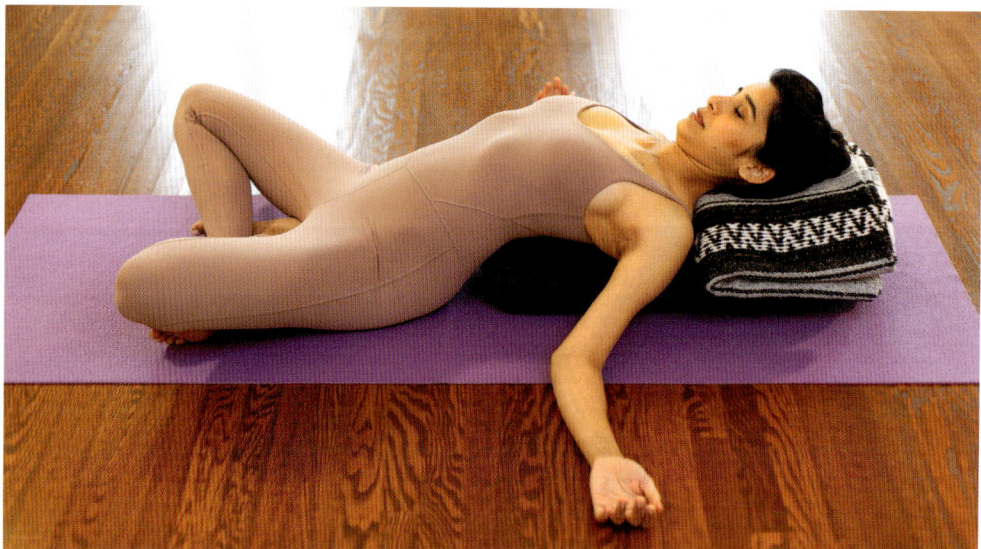

FIGURE 2.14.  **Supta Swastikāsana**

## 5. Adho Mukha Swastikāsana (Downward-Facing Crossed Legs)

Sit on one or two folded blankets in Swastikāsana with your legs crossed, feet directly under your knees. Sit toward the front edge of the blankets and lift the spine. Those with more mobility in the hips may find it more grounding to sit directly on the floor. Fold forward from the hips and rest your forehead on a blanket or bolster, placed across the seat of a chair. Cross your forearms overhead and rest them on the support. Keep the sides of your waist and abdomen lifted and the shoulder blades moving down your back (fig. 2.15). Soften the groins and spread the buttock bones and the pelvic floor muscles. You may feel the spreading action in the pelvic floor muscles more clearly as they make contact with the blanket. Stay for one to two minutes, then come up and repeat with the alternate cross of the legs.

Note that students with more mobility may find that they can easily move the head lower on the seat of the chair. However, those who are stiff or newly postpartum should take care not to compress the abdomen or round the spine, which can put pressure on the pelvic organs. If any compression or dropping of the chest is felt, or strain in the neck, increase the height of the head support by adding folded blankets or a bolster.

**Effects:** *This supported forward bend soothes backache, removes stiffness in the hips, and helps the pelvic floor muscles spread. It also quiets the mind and nervous system and helps relieve fatigue.*

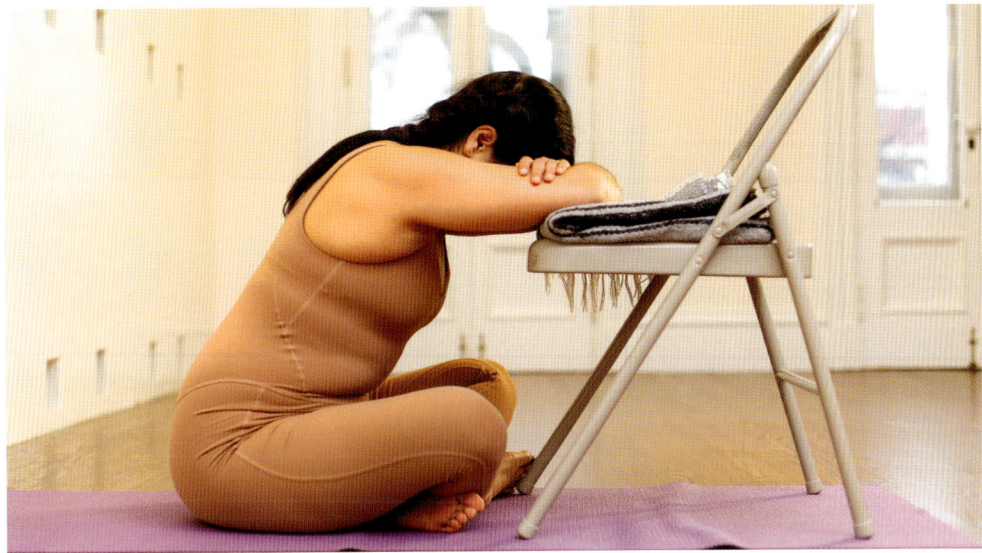

FIGURE 2.15. **Adho Mukha Swastikāsana**

### 6. ADHO MUKHA VĪRĀSANA (DOWNWARD-FACING HERO'S POSE)

Sit on your heels with your knees apart. If the buttocks don't reach the heels, or if you have knee pain, place a folded blanket or two between the buttocks and the heels. Have a bolster and narrow folded blanket directly in front of you, and pull the bolster and blanket close to you between your thighs. Maintaining the press of the buttocks toward the heels, lift your abdomen and fold forward over the bolster, resting the abdomen and torso completely on the bolster. For larger bodies or for those with less range of motion in the knees and hips, a second bolster can be added to better support the torso. Rest your forehead on the support or, alternatively, roll a blanket under your forehead for easier breathing. Fold or roll a blanket under your forehead and rest your forehead. Stretch your arms forward, lengthening the sides of your waist and side chest forward. Gently continue to stretch the spine forward while resting the brain completely on the rolled blanket. Keep pressing your hips back, but allow the buttock bones to spread away from each other. Continue breathing in the manner described previously, inhaling while relaxing and spreading the pelvic floor.

More than any other pose in this sequence, you may feel a dramatic spreading action in the pelvic floor on the inhalation. This pose can be very useful for those who have high tonicity in the pelvic muscles. Pay attention to the exhalation and notice whether there are any clenching or contracting reactions. If so, try to release the pelvic floor muscles with each inhalation and gradually resist the urge to clench. Over time, you may find that you gain better control over these movements and that over-clenching diminishes.

**Effects:** *This supported forward bend softens and spreads the pelvic floor and removes stiffness in the hips and fatigue in the lower back. It is deeply soothing for the nervous system and quiets a busy mind.*

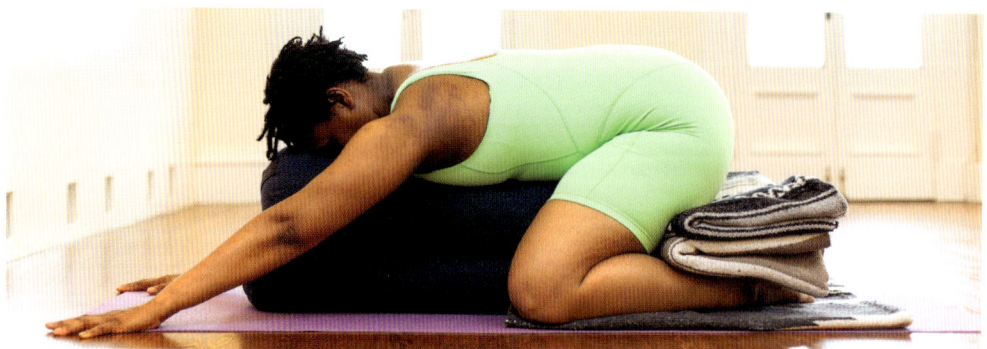

FIGURE 2.16. **Adho Mukha Vīrāsana**

## 7. Setubandha Sarvāṅgāsana (Supported Bridge Pose)

Setubandha is a wonderful postpartum pose, but some experimenting may be needed to find the best setup for you. We have intentionally kept the following setups simple and accessible.

Sit on the edge of a bolster on a smooth floor, with no mat, facing the wall. Place a block at the medium height at the wall. Lie back and slide your shoulders off the bolster until the tops of your shoulders come down to touch the floor. See that the back of your head, neck, and both arms are fully resting on the floor. Stretch your legs out one at a time, resting your heels on the block, soles of your feet at the wall (fig. 2.17). If the knees are bent, press your feet into the wall and slide the bolster back away from the wall to extend your legs fully, moving carefully so your chest does not slide off the bolster. Extend the buttocks toward the heels and lengthen the side ribs toward the crown of your head in order to lengthen and gently stretch the abdomen. With your chin moving toward your chest, soften your throat and face.

### VARIATIONS

All students may belt the legs at the mid- or upper thighs or the shins, ankles, or outer feet for more compactness and stability in the legs and pelvis. For newly postpartum people, if belting the legs together causes you to lose the inward movement of the tailbone, then start with the legs slightly apart, and slowly work toward taking them together (fig. 2.18). Additionally,

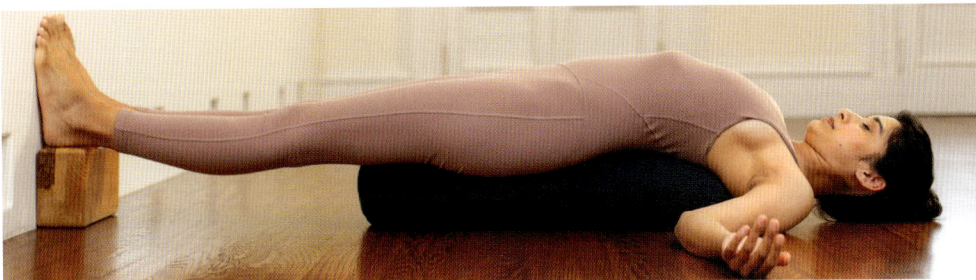

FIGURE 2.17. Setubandha Sarvāṅgāsana, feet on blocks.

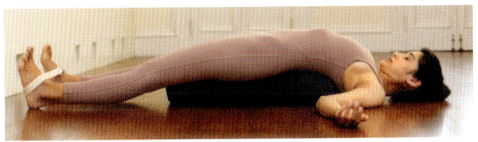

FIGURE 2.18. Feet belted

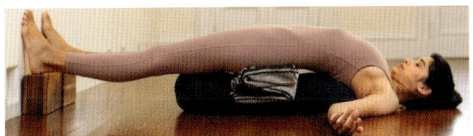

FIGURE 2.19. Additional height under pelvis

you can place a block between the upper thighs, belting around the thighs to create both compactness in the hips and spreading in the inner groins, pelvis, and abdomen (fig. 2.20).

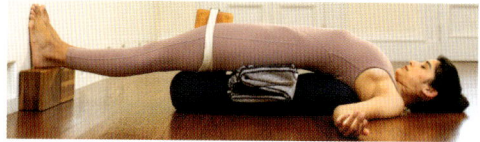

FIGURE 2.20. **Block between thighs, thighs belted**

BACKACHE: Place a folded blanket under your sacrum and buttocks to elevate the pelvis and bring the tailbone in (fig. 2.19). Keep your legs hips width apart on two blocks, with or without belts. This variation gives more lift to the pelvis and helps support the pelvic organs. Those with large or wide hips or buttocks or a strong lumbar curve may need a wider support. Place two blocks at their medium height on either side of the bolster, with a triple-folded blanket on top

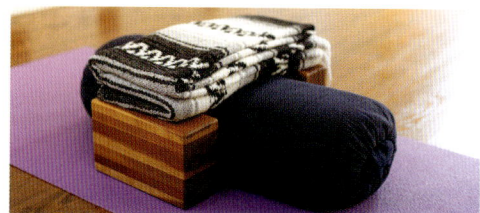

FIGURE 2.21. **Setup for Fig 2.22**

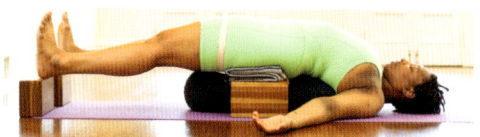

FIGURE 2.22. **Two blocks and triple-folded blanket under pelvis**

of the bolster and both bricks (figs. 2.21 and 2.22). You should now have a "saddle" for the pelvis, with the blocks slightly higher than the bolster. This variation helps lift the outer hips and rolls the hip bones inward, creating a soft cradling action for the organs.

NECK PAIN OR TIGHT SHOULDERS: If the upper back is stiff, add a flat blanket under the shoulders and head or a rolled blanket under the neck.

*Effects:* *This supported inversion aerates the organs and abdominal muscles with fresh blood as well as opens the chest and lungs. It quiets the mind and nervous system and helps to stimulate and balance the endocrine system.*

### 8. Viparīta Karaṇī with Bent Legs (Reversed-Action Pose or Legs-Up-the-Wall Pose)

Place a bolster horizontally in front of a chair. Sit sideways on the bolster and lie back as you swing your legs onto the seat of the chair. Your sacrum should be well supported by the bolster. Adjust the distance of the chair so that your calves are spreading and the backs of your knees are hooked on the edge of the

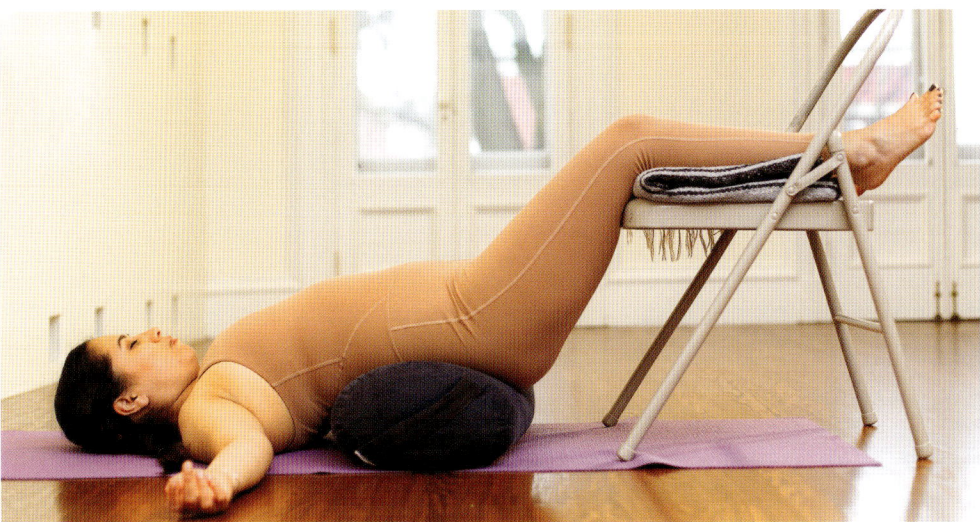

FIGURE 2.23. **Viparīta Karaṇī with bent legs.**

chair (you may have to move the chair back). Rest your legs completely, using one or two folded blankets on the chair seat to support your calves and the backs of your knees. Keep your shoulder blades moving down your back and turn your palms up to keep the top chest open. Soften and spread the abdomen as you simultaneously spread the lumbar spinal muscles laterally. Move your eyes away from each other and soften the skin on your face, resting the face completely. Use longer exhalations to cultivate overall quietness of the body and mind.

**Effects:** *This supported inversion releases tension in the lumbar spine, hips, and abdomen. It creates softening in the groins and abdomen and teaches the relaxation of the pelvic floor muscles. Additionally, it relieves fatigue, quiets the mind, and brings serenity to the whole nervous system.*

## 9. ŚAVĀSANA (CORPSE POSE)

Lie flat with your legs and arms resting evenly away from the midline. Move the flesh of your buttocks toward your heels so that the lower spine is lengthened. Turn your upper arms from the inside out to spread the chest. Move your top shoulders down your back and lengthen the back of your skull away from your neck to create quietness in the throat. Support your head and neck with a folded blanket if needed. As you breathe, continue to soften your abdomen, pelvic floor muscles, face, tongue, and eyes. Breathe softly and rhythmically. On the inhalation, softly spread the pelvic floor muscles. On the exhalation, feel a slight lift and return of those muscles. Take care not to push or contract unnecessarily. The focus should be on observation. Notice whether the awareness and softening effect of your pelvic floor has increased from the beginning of the sequence.

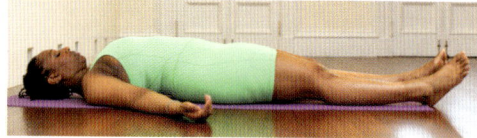

FIGURE 2.24.  Śavāsana

### VARIATIONS

BACKACHE: Do Śavāsana with the spine flat and the legs supported on a chair, or tuck a bolster under your knees.

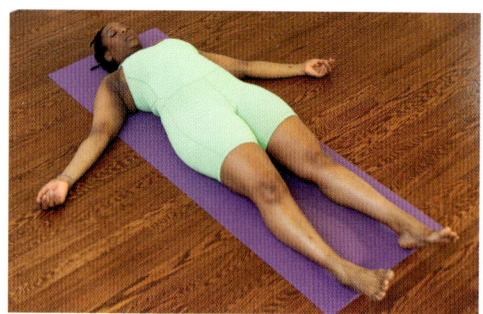

FIGURE 2.25.  Śavāsana, alternate view

*Effects:* *Śavāsana is the time when the whole body can rest and the actions from the previous āsanas are integrated into the body. It relieves fatigue and anxiety and brings a calming and cooling effect to the whole body and mind.*

## WEEK 1 FULL SEQUENCE

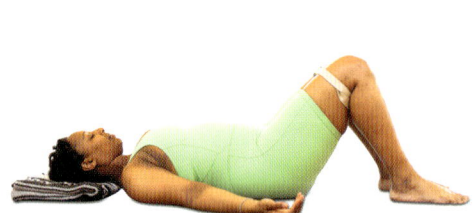

1.  **Establishing your breath** (page 55)

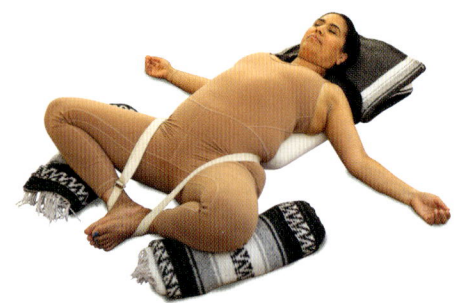

2.  **Supta Baddha Koṇāsana** (page 56)

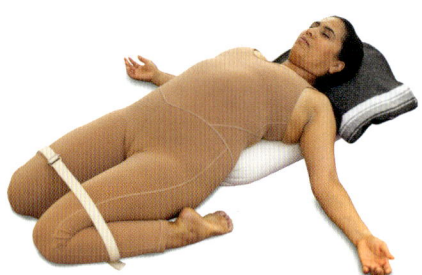

3.  **Supta Vīrāsana** (page 58)

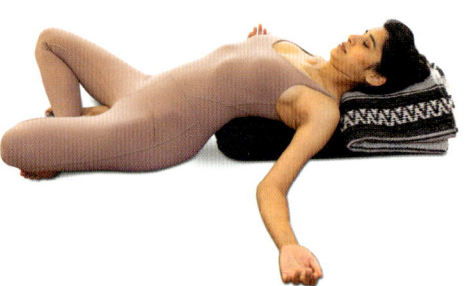

4.  **Supta Swastikāsana** (page 60)

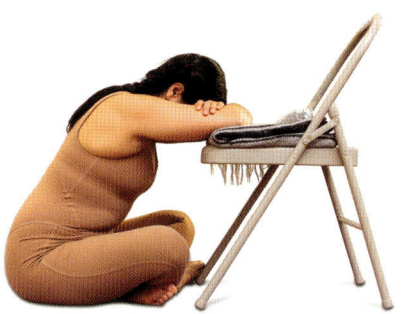

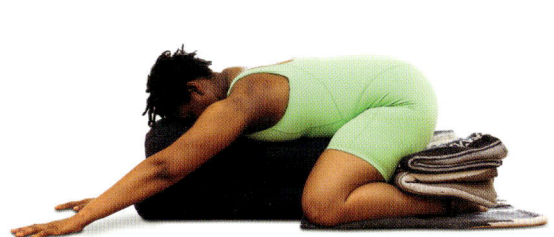

5. **Adho Mukha Swastikāsana (page 61)**

6. **Adho Mukha Vīrāsana (page 62)**

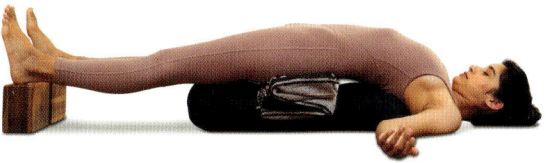

7. **Setubandha Sarvāṅgāsana (page 63)**

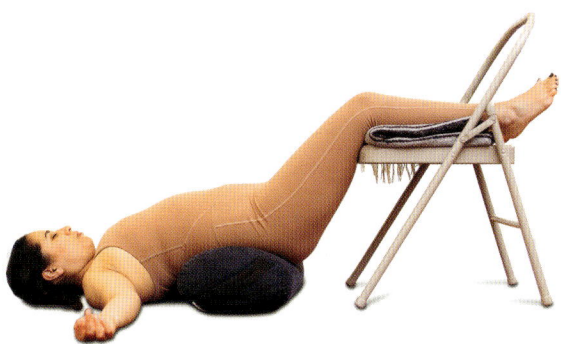

8. **Viparīta Karaṇī, legs bent (page 65)**

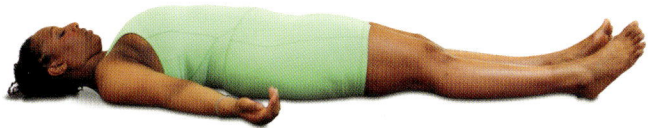

9. **Śavāsana (page 65)**

# Week 2
# MOVING TOWARD PELVIC ALIGNMENT

Hopefully by now you've begun to establish a connection with your pelvic floor, noticing the rhythm of your breath in conjunction with the movements of the muscles. Once you've begun to connect with and feel the movements of your pelvic floor through your breath, you may begin to notice areas of tension, numbness, pain, or imbalance in the pelvic floor. This is a common experience for most practitioners and an important part of getting to know your own "landscape." If we can approach these areas of difficulty or imbalance slowly, with curiosity, and with an experiential intention, we can start to unravel what are most often multilayered and sometimes chronic challenges.

As we move into the next sequence of āsanas, we begin to make mild adjustments to the legs, hips, sacrum, and lower spine to help bring optimum alignment to the pelvis and pelvic organs and to set the stage for later pelvic floor strengthening. We begin to notice the relationship between the top, bottom, and sides of the pelvis. In particular, we focus on how the legs help support the pelvis when we stand. We notice the relationship between the pubis and coccyx (see "Bony Anatomy of the Pelvis" in chapter 1) and how to adjust the position of the pelvis so the organs inside are supported.

As you start to make adjustments, take care to maintain the relaxation of the pelvic floor muscles acquired in the previous sequence. As we now learn to release tension even in standing or inverted āsanas, it's important to maintain the relaxation of the pelvic floor with the in-breath. If, on the other hand, you find that you're not ready for the poses in this sequence, or you can't maintain the awareness and relaxation found previously, it's better to return to the poses that helped you gain maximum relaxation and ease in your breath. We encourage you to go slowly, without straining, paying attention to any pain or restriction. If in doubt, back off, or return to an easier pose so that you can maintain that vital connection and awareness to your pelvic floor. Once you begin feeling stable and confident in these Week 2 poses, you may start to notice a feeling of lift or lightness. As you go through this week's sequence, here are some guiding questions to keep in mind:

Can I retain the release of the pelvic floor muscles with my inhalation?

Do I feel my pelvic floor lifting with my exhalation, without gripping?

Do I feel supported by the actions of my legs in the āsanas?

Postpartum people can begin this sequence once bleeding has completely stopped. However, in the case of extreme fatigue, you should start with Sālamba Sarvāṅgāsana, which can be practiced alone or in the middle of the previous sequence between Adho Mukha Swastikāsana and Setubandha Sarvāṅgāsana; then, gradually add the standing poses over a few weeks. If you have had a cesarean delivery, you should wait eight weeks or until obtaining approval from your doctor before beginning these āsanas. These poses can be practiced during menstruation, with the exception of Sālamba Sarvāṅgāsana and Ardha Hālāsana.

## Sequence of Āsanas: Week 2

### 1. TĀḌĀSANA WITH A BLOCK (MOUNTAIN POSE)

Stand with your feet hips width apart and place a block at its narrow width as high up between your thighs as possible, making sure the front and sides of the block are even. Keeping your inner heels and balls of the feet firmly pressing into the mat, lift from the inner arches to the inner knees to the inner thighs to lift the block upward. Draw the outer shin bones and thigh bones in toward the midline and bring your tailbone forward toward the base of the pubis while pressing the fronts of your thighs back. Keep the bottom of the

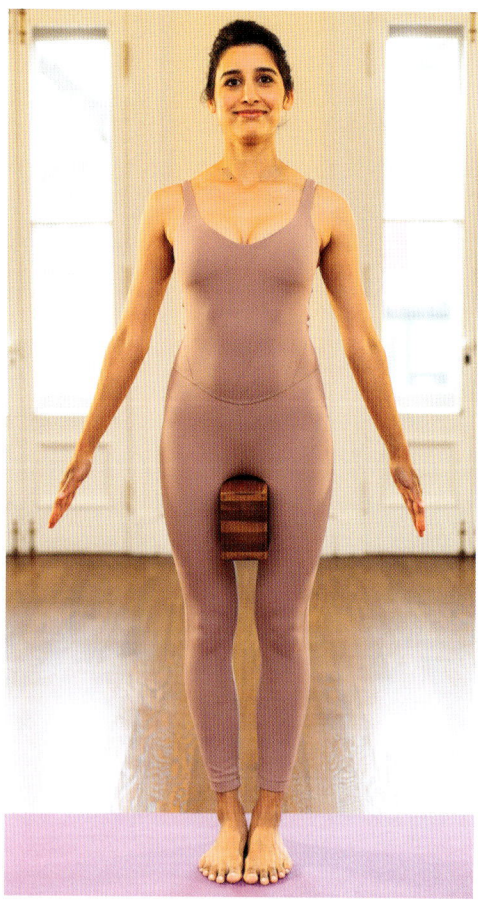

FIGURE 2.26. **Tāḍāsana with a block.**

pubis moving toward the tailbone, but lift the top of the pubis up toward your navel. Lift and spread your navel and spread the diaphragm. Notice whether the inner thighs are doing all the work. If so, relax the inner legs slightly and hug the block from the outer thighs, feeling the spreading effect on your pelvis and abdomen. Feel how the leg work allows the spine to lift organically. Lift and spread your chest as you stretch down through your arms. Relax your face and throat and let your eyes be quiet.

To intensify the effect of the leg work on the spine, belt your hip sockets, middle thighs, and center of the shin bones. This allows for further groin, pelvic floor, and abdominal softening. An additional block can be placed between your knees for better leg alignment.

**Effects:** *This standing pose energizes and aligns the legs and teaches the legs to support the pelvis and pelvic floor muscles. The block provides feedback to the pelvic floor muscles to spread while also beginning to lift. It also teaches the correct alignment of the tailbone moving toward the pubis.*

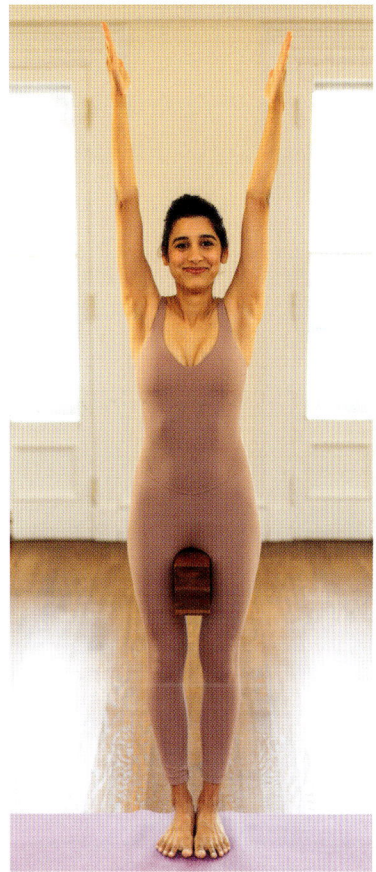

FIGURE 2.27.  **Ūrdhva Hastāsana**

## 2. ŪRDHVA HASTĀSANA (UPWARD STRETCHED HANDS)

From Tāḍāsana, move your arms up with the palms facing each other. Lift the sides of your waist and straighten your arms, keeping your elbows firm. Use your arms to lift the whole of your spine higher away from the block. Continue to move the tailbone in while pressing your thighs back. As you stretch your arms upward, observe the tailbone and pubis alignment—the block should not swing forward or backward. Keep your lumbar spine

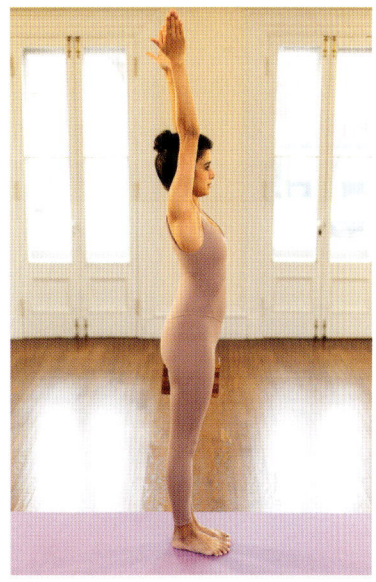

FIGURE 2.28.  **Side view**

lifted and your lower ribs moving back so your abdomen doesn't get pushed forward. If the abdominal-lumbar action is lost, the pelvic organs will become compressed, in which case, lower your arms, realign your pelvis, and then stretch your arms up again. This can be repeated a few times.

**Effects** *This pose further elongates and energizes the spine. The actions of the arms serve to stretch the shoulders and bring lightness and vitality to the chest, relieving fatigue.*

### 3. Ūrdhva Baddhanguliyāsana (Upward Bound Fingers)

From Tāḍāsana, interlock your fingers, turn your palms inside out, and stretch your arms upward. Keeping your elbows firm, move your arms

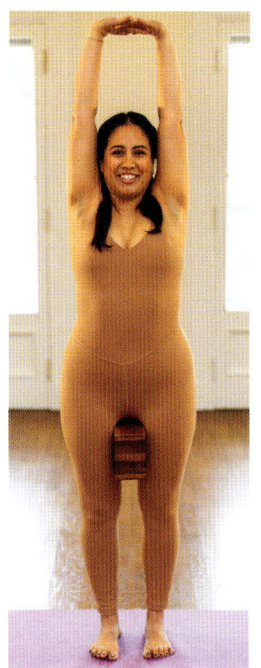
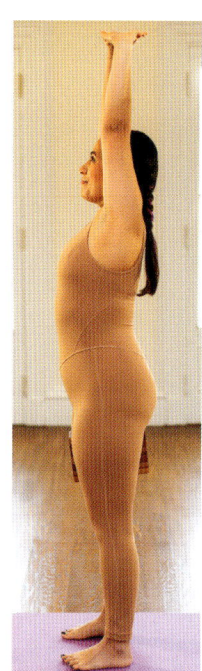

FIGURE 2.29. **Ūrdhva Baddhanguliyāsana**

FIGURE 2.30. **Side view**

back toward your ears and open your armpits. Keep your shoulder blades spreading and keep your neck and throat soft. Maintain your leg actions from Tāḍāsana as you further lift your back ribs up and spread your diaphragm. This variation can be repeated a few times to ensure proper pelvic alignment.

**Effects** *This arm action opens the shoulder girdle and helps lift the back ribs and the back of the diaphragm, bringing more breath and space to the chest.*

### 4. Ardha Uttānāsana with a Block (Half Intense Stretch)

Place a block at its narrow width as high up between your thighs as possible. Now face the wall and walk back with your fingertips on the wall (the block can be inserted after walking back if it is difficult). Straighten your arms, legs, and spine, adjusting the distance from the wall so that your hips are directly over your heels and

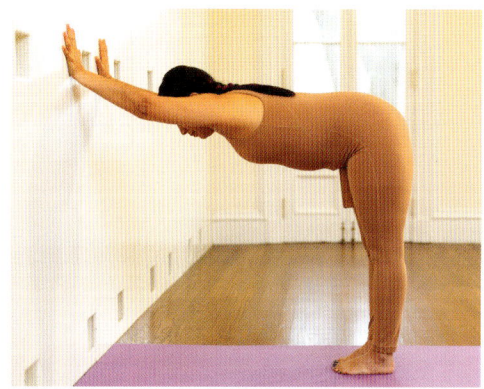

FIGURE 2.31. **Ardha Uttānāsana**

your trunk is parallel to the floor. Lift the inner arches of your feet, your inner knees, and your inner thighs, pressing the block back to move the inner groins back. Feel the inner rotation of your inner thighs and lift and spread the backs of your thighs and buttocks. Spread the pelvic floor muscles. Press your fingers into the wall, keep your elbows firm, and move your hips back to lengthen your side trunk. Watch that your abdomen doesn't push down to the floor; rather, gently lift your abdomen toward your spine. Keep your head and neck in line with your upper arms and breathe into the side lungs.

**Effects** *This standing pose stretches the backs of your thighs and buttocks, creating freedom in the pelvis and space for the pelvic floor muscles to spread. It elongates the spine and opens the shoulders, bringing energy to the whole body. In addition, it gently tones the abdominal organs toward the spine.*

### 5. Pārśvottānāsana with a Foot on a Block (Intense Side-Stretch Pose)

Angle a block vertically at 45 degrees against the wall. Face the wall. With your hands supported on the wall, step your right foot forward and step your left foot back. Angle your front foot so that your heel is on the floor and the ball of your foot is up on the block (fig. 2.32). Step the back foot farther back—about four to four and a half feet—and angle your toes about 45 degrees from the edge of the mat. Straighten your legs fully. While maintaining the outer edge of your back

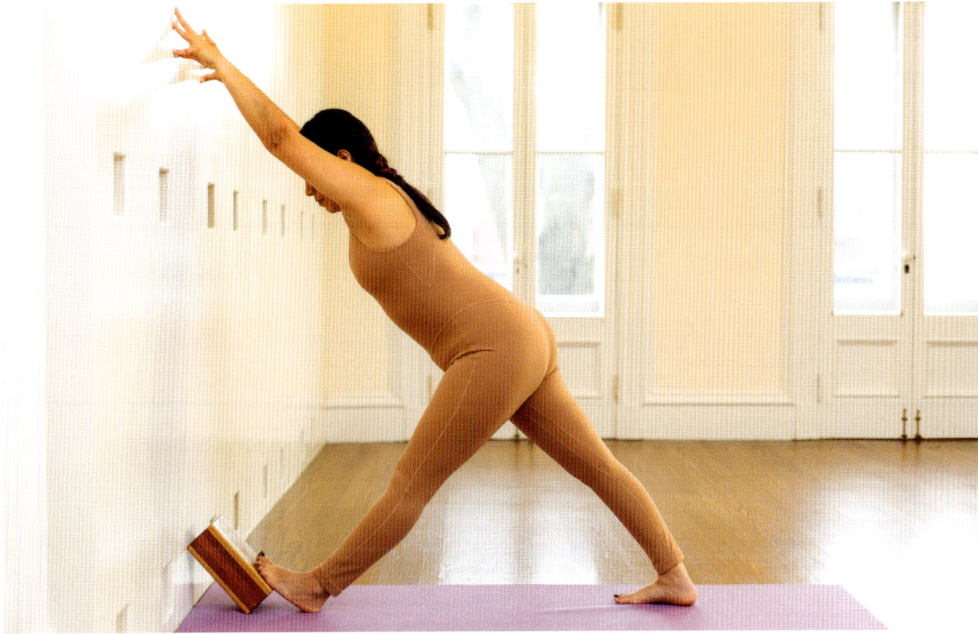

FIGURE 2.32. **Pārśvottānāsana**

heel firmly pressing into the floor, revolve the back of your back thigh so the back hip comes forward in line with your front hip. See that the hips are evenly facing the wall. Press the inner ball mound of your front foot down on the block but keep the inner arch lifting. You can lift your toes to help initiate this action. Keep your knees and thighs engaged and lifted. Draw your front-leg hip back and in toward the midline, compacting your hips. Maintain this action as you walk your hands higher up the wall, stretching the sides of your waist up

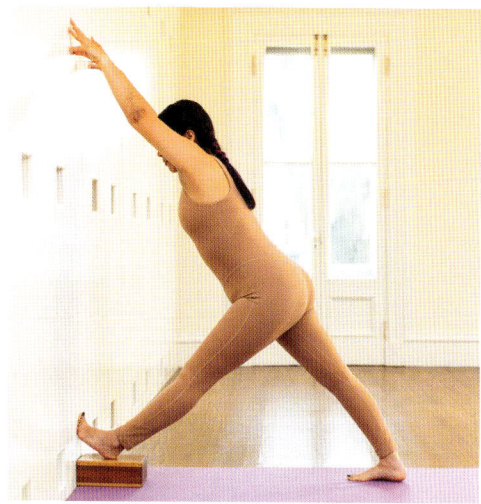

FIGURE 2.33. **Foot on a block at the wall**

strongly. To come out, walk your hands down, and step your back foot forward and your front foot back. Then repeat on the other side.

## VARIATIONS

THOSE WHO ARE NEWLY POSTPARTUM: Ideally, the heel of the front foot should be in line with the back arch. However, you may benefit from taking your legs more widely apart initially so that the abdominal organs maintain their spreading. Over time, the legs can be brought closer together.

INTENSIFYING THE POSE: Place the block at its lowest aspect, flat on the floor. Move your heel up on the block with the ball of your foot pressing the wall (fig. 2.33). This intensifies the effects of the pose.

*Effects This standing pose stretches the legs, spine, and arms while teaching the compacting action of the hips. Many people, especially those who are post-partum, experience hip instability in conjunction with pelvic floor weakness or dysfunction. The foot on the block creates strengthening actions in the front leg and helps to move the thigh bone back into the hip socket, bringing proper align-ment to the hips. These hip actions, in conjunction with the lift and stretch of the arms and chest, helps the pelvic and abdominal organs to lift and get gently toned toward the spine. The current of energy begins to move upward from the pelvic floor to the chest (prāṇa vāyu), which is especially beneficial after the downward moving energy of childbirth (apāna vāyu).*

### 6. Sālamba Sarvāṅgāsana (Supported All-Limbed Pose or Shoulder Stand)

Sālamba Sarvāṅgāsana is presented in stages to ensure that even a beginner student can attempt the pose safely. Even advanced practitioners who are recovering from childbirth and pregnancy, or other pelvic or abdominal trauma, may find that practicing the beginning stages of the pose for some time is beneficial for healing. Here, a basic setup is shown so that beginners can practice the pose with minimal props. Before you begin, look through all the stages as well as the next pose, Hālāsana, so that you can set up accordingly.

### STAGE 1. BENT LEGS

Stack three blankets with the round folded edge in line with the short edge of the mat. Fold the tail end of the mat halfway over the blankets. Position this entire setup about 6 to 10 inches away from the wall with the folded edges of the blankets facing away from the wall. Lie down with your buttocks against the wall, shoulders on the edge of the blankets, and head on the floor. The shoulders should be **on the blankets,** close to the edge of the blankets, but not falling off. If your buttocks are too far from the wall, or your shoulders are falling off the blankets, get up and reposition the whole setup before attempting the pose.

Once you have adjusted to the correct distance, lie down, bend your knees, and place your feet on the wall. Stretch your arms toward the wall, grab the outer edge of the mat, and turn your upper arms from inside out to open your armpits. Simultaneously press your outer upper arms down, press your feet into the wall, and raise your buttocks up. In coming into the pose, take care to not push your shoulders off the blankets. Now bend your elbows and place your hands on your back ribs. Walk your hands farther down your back toward the shoulder blades and strongly lift your back ribs up. Imagine that you are dragging the wall down with your feet (without actually moving your

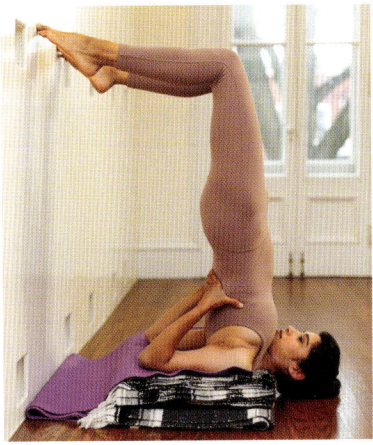

**FIGURE 2.34.  Sālamba Sarvāṅgāsana with bent legs.**

feet) as you lift your buttocks up. Firm your buttocks, draw your hamstrings in toward the buttocks, and lift your buttocks higher. Now come onto the tips of your toes and raise your tailbone strongly upward toward the ceiling. Your spine should be perpendicular to the floor with your legs at a right angle. If your knees are too far back (the wall feels too far away), it is better to come down and move the blankets closer to the wall, as too much arching of your back puts strain on your abdomen. Stay for one to three minutes, or to your capacity, and then release your hands and come down.

**Effects** *This stage of Sarvāṅgāsana firms the buttock muscles and helps bring the tailbone in, lengthening the iliopsoas and quadriceps muscles, which is especially helpful for those with an anterior tilt in the pelvis, as is common after pregnancy. The spine lifts and the abdominal organs and muscles are gently tonified. The entire pelvis is inverted, and the organs now work with gravity rather than against it. You may feel immediate relief from pelvic organ prolapse and heaviness. Additionally, the thyroid, parathyroid, and pituitary glands are stimulated, helping to balance the endocrine system. With some practice, Sarvāṅgāsana brings deep relief to the nervous system and quiets the mind.*

You should practice stage 1 (bent legs) until your pelvis can be lifted perpendicular to the floor while keeping your buttocks firm. Once that is established, you can move on to stage 2. If you are postpartum, you may need to practice this stage for several weeks until you feel stable enough to move to the next stage.

## STAGE 2. ALTERNATING LEGS

Start in stage 1 (bent legs). Keeping your left toes on the wall, raise your right leg up toward the ceiling. Straighten your right leg fully, keep both sides of the pelvis lifting evenly, and maintain the action of your tailbone ascending upward (fig. 2.35). Bring your right foot back to the wall and repeat on the left. Observe how the pelvis and pelvic floor muscles respond as you extend each leg upward.

You should practice stage 2 until your pelvis can maintain its evenness and your tailbone and buttocks are lifting well when one leg is raised. Once that is established, you can move on to stage 3.

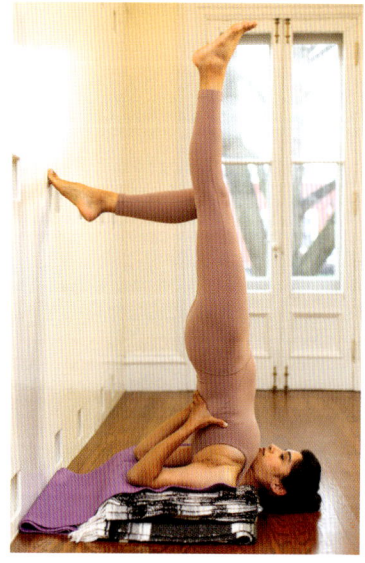

FIGURE 2.35. **Alternating legs**

## STAGE 3. FULL POSE

Start in stage 1, with your knees bent and both feet on the wall. Now, take one foot and then the other off the wall, stretching your legs straight upward (figs. 2.36 and 2.37). At first, the buttocks may fall onto your hands. Lift your buttocks up strongly toward your heels and walk your hands farther down toward the shoulder blades to lift the back ribs up again. Stretch up from your buttocks to your heels and open the backs of your knees. Roll your thighs inward and spread the backs of your thighs, keeping your tailbone moving strongly into your body. At first, it may be difficult to bring your legs together. If the tailbone and buttock actions are lost when you move your legs together, start with your feet hip distance apart and gradually bring your legs together over time. To come out, one at a time bring your feet back to the wall, release your hands, and lower your trunk down. Rest there for a short while.

## VARIATIONS

Once you are able to practice these three stages confidently, the following props may be helpful:

- Belt the upper elbows, shoulder width apart, in order to keep your elbows from splaying out and to help lift your chest.

- Place a block between your upper thighs, as in Tāḍāsana, described in pose 1, and tie a belt around your hip sockets, middle thighs, shins, or ankles (fig. 2.38). This gives a similar effect as in Tāḍāsana: the inner thighs and groins soften, and the outer hips become compact. However, in the inversion, the pelvic floor receives an even greater spreading action, while simultaneously the pelvic organs move back to their proper place.

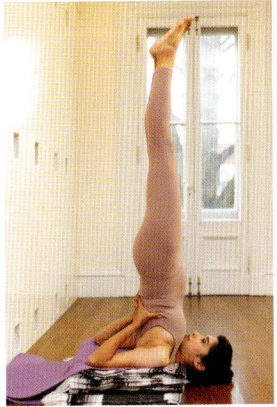

**FIGURE 2.36.** **Full pose, side view**

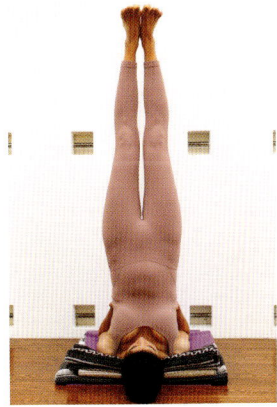

**FIGURE 2.37.** **Full pose, front view**

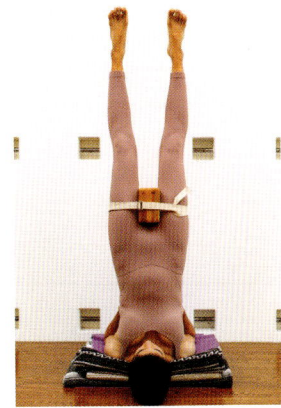

**FIGURE 2.38.** **Variation with a block between the thighs, legs belted**

• Tie a belt or resistance band around the outer edges of your feet (the outer metatarsals) about hips width apart (fig. 2.39). Press your feet out into the belt in order to suck the femur heads into the sockets. This is especially good for hip joint instability as it activates the medial gluteus muscles and other abductors.

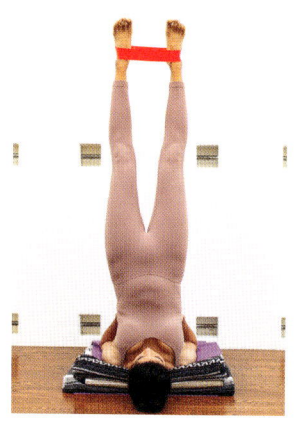

**FIGURE 2.39.** Variation with a resistance band on the outer feet

### 7. ARDHA HĀLĀSANA (HALF PLOW POSE)

Before attempting Ardha Hālāsana, you should feel confident balancing in Sarvāṅgāsana (pose 6, fig 2.36), at least momentarily. You will be coming into Ardha Hālāsana from Sarvāṅgāsana.

Position a chair two feet away from the rounded edge of your Sarvāṅgāsana blankets, toward the head side. Start in Sarvāṅgāsana. Keeping your upper arms firmly pressing into the floor and your hands supporting the back ribs, lower your legs down to the chair one at a time (fig. 2.40). Keep your legs active: press your toes and the ball mounds of your feet down into the chair seat as you raise your knees and thighs upward, sucking the muscles to the bones. Walk your hands farther down toward the shoulder blades and lift your back ribs up. Lift your hips up and grow the spine long. Release the back of your neck away from your shoulders and let the chin soften toward your chest, relaxing your throat. Soften and rest your eyes. The abdomen should be lifted and soft. If the abdomen is compressed, or the spine is rounding, raise

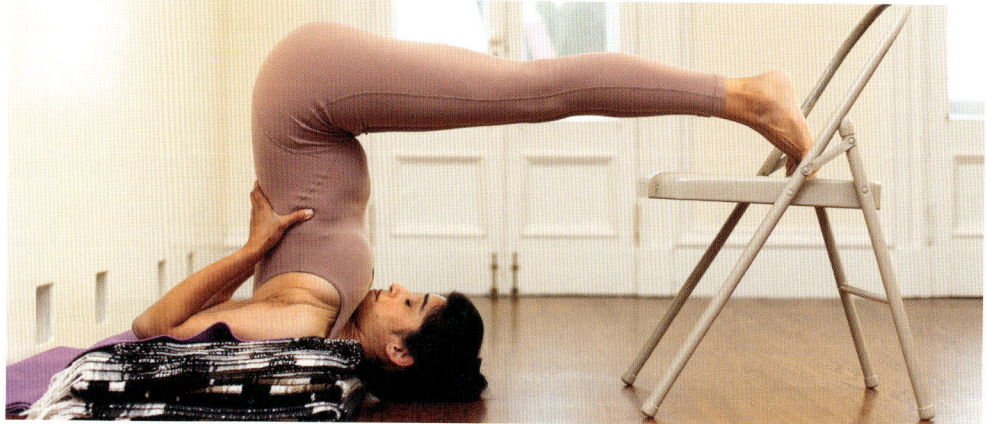

**FIGURE 2.40.** Hālāsana, feet on chair

your feet higher by adding blocks or a bolster on the chair. Stay for one to two minutes, or to your capacity, then raise your legs back up and return to Sarvāṅgāsana. To come down, put your feet on the wall one at a time, release your hands, and lower down. Rest there for some time.

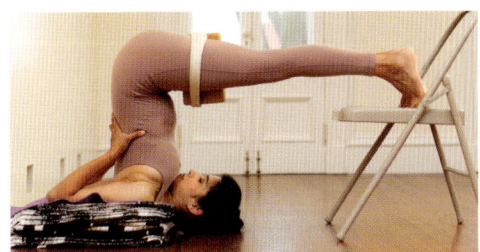

**FIGURE 2.41.** **Variation with a block between the thighs, legs belted**

**Effects** *This inversion stimulates the thyroid and parathyroid glands and soothes the vagus nerve, bringing deep relaxation.*

## VARIATIONS

- As in the previous pose, Sālamba Sarvāṅgāsana, place a block between the thighs and belt the thighs for a similar effect.

### 8. Supta Baddha Koṇāsana with a Cone

Fold a mat in quarters. Holding one corner of the mat in place with one hand, use your other hand to roll a cone from the corner of the opposite side (fig. 2.42). Sit on your rolled mat, a few inches in front of the edge of the tip of the cone. When you lie down, the tip of the cone should be under your lower back. The tip will face toward the head side and the wide tail of the cone will be between your legs. Bring your feet to Baddha Koṇāsana, with your feet up on the wide part of the cone and your heels close to the groins. If that is difficult, place your feet under the wide

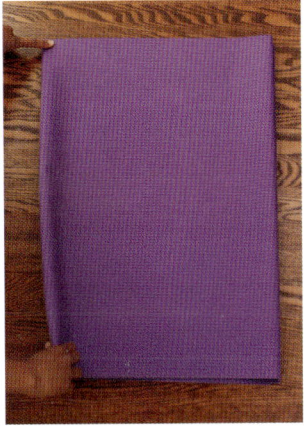
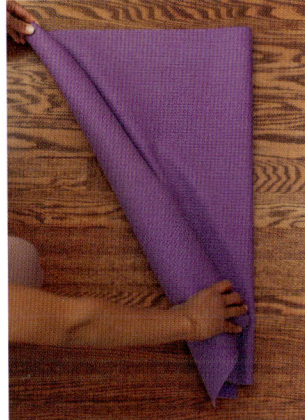
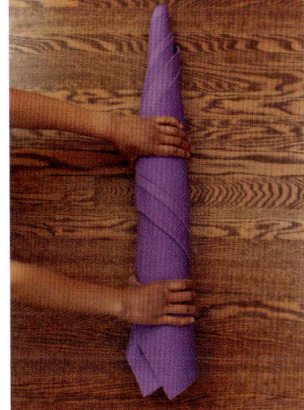

**FIGURE 2.42.** **Rolling the cone**

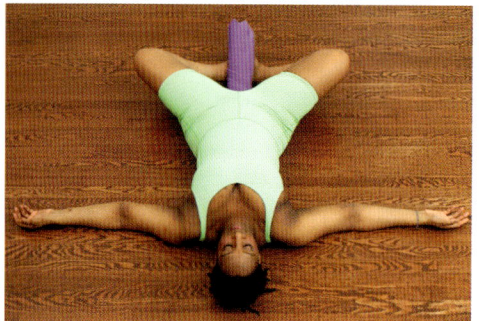

FIGURE 2.43. **Feet under the cone**

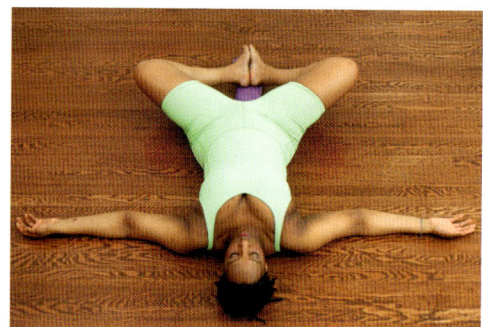

FIGURE 2.44. **Feet on top of the cone**

part of the cone. Press your heels gently to spread your inner thighs. Now, slowly slide your lumbar spine off the cone so that the lumbar spine lengthens away from your buttocks, and the pubis moves toward your navel. The tip of the cone should now be under your tailbone. Alternately, have a helper pull the wide tail of the cone away from you to draw the buttocks away from the lumbar, creating greater traction. Let your abdomen relax and soften. Relax your arms, throat, and face. Breathe slowly, softening and spreading the pelvic floor on the inhalation.

## VARIATIONS

This pose can be practiced flat on the floor, as shown in figures 2.43 and 2.44, in order to feel the actions of your tailbone and pubis. Some postpartum people may feel a soothing effect in the lower back from being flat on the floor but may need to add the additional support of blankets under the thighs.

Once the effects of the cone can be felt, try using the cone in the fully supported version of Supta Baddha Koṇāsana, shown in Week 1, pose 2. The cone can also be used with other supine poses like Supta Vīrāsana and Supta Swastikāsana, as well as in Setubandha Sarvāṅgāsana (see Week 1 for instructions on these poses). Notice, for example, the positive effect of the cone on the position of the pelvis and abdomen in Setubandha in figures 2.45 and 2.46 below.

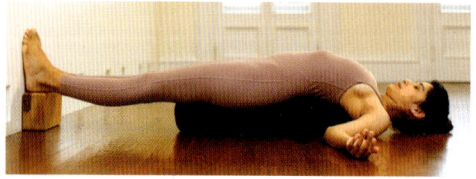

FIGURE 2.45. **Setubandha Sarvāṅgāsana with no cone**

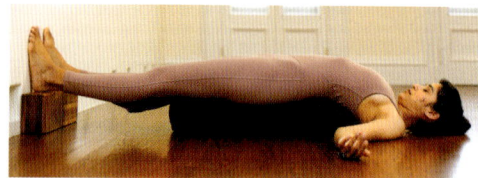

FIGURE 2.46. **Setubandha Sarvāṅgāsana with the cone**

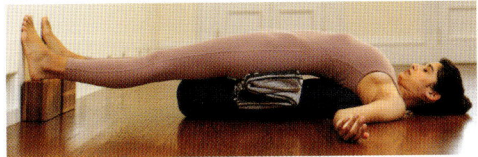

FIGURE 2.47. Setubandha Sarvāṅgāsana

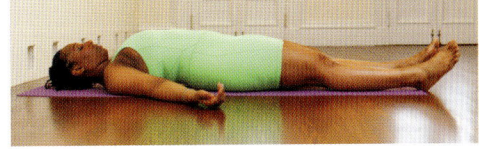

FIGURE 2.48. Śavāsana

**Effects** *The cone helps the tailbone to move in and corrects anterior tilting of the pelvis. The abdomen becomes soft and the spine becomes a "bed" for the organs.*

After practicing Supta Baddha Koṇāsana, you may continue with the rest of the Week 1 āsanas, or proceed to:

## 9. SETUBANDHA SARVĀṄGĀSANA

See fig. 2.47 and Week 1 pose 7 for instructions.

## 10. ŚAVĀSANA

See fig. 2.48 and Week 1 pose 9 for instructions.

## WEEK 2 FULL SEQUENCE

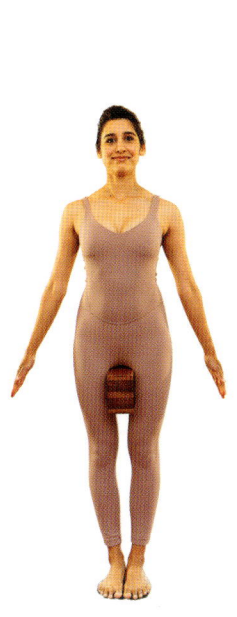

1. Tāḍāsana with block (page 70)

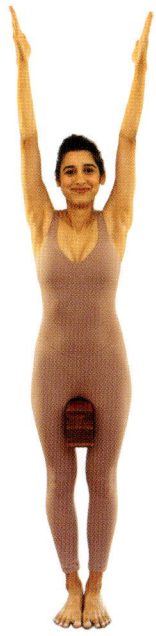

2. Ūrdhva Hast-āsana (page 71)

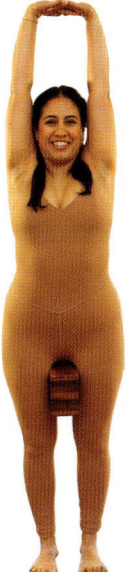

3. Ūrdhva Baddhanguli-yāsana (page 72)

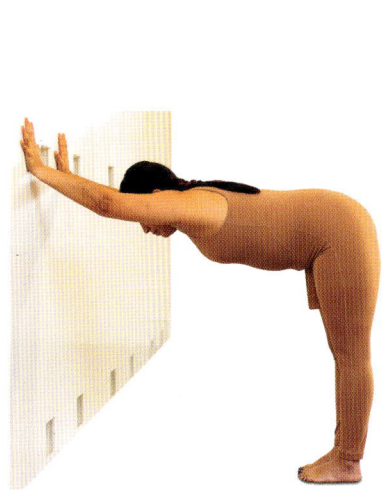

4. Ardha Uttānāsana (page 72)

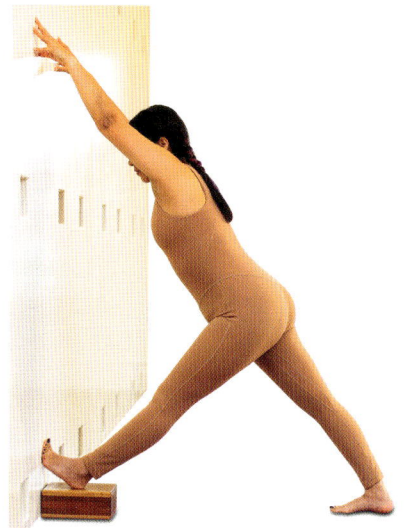

5. Pārśvottānāsana (page 73)

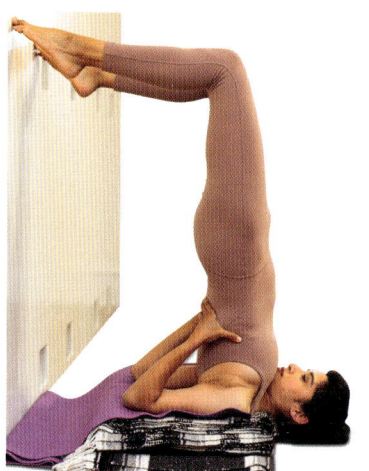

6. Sālamba Sarvāṅgāsana (page 75)

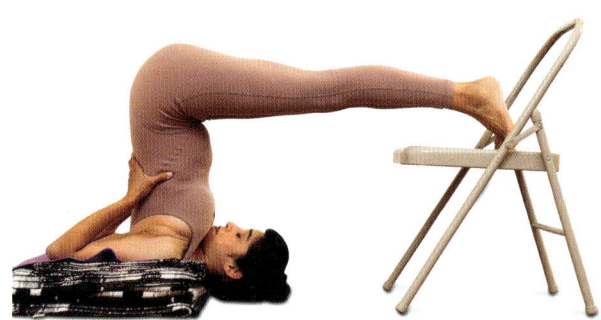

7. Ardha Hālāsana (page 78)

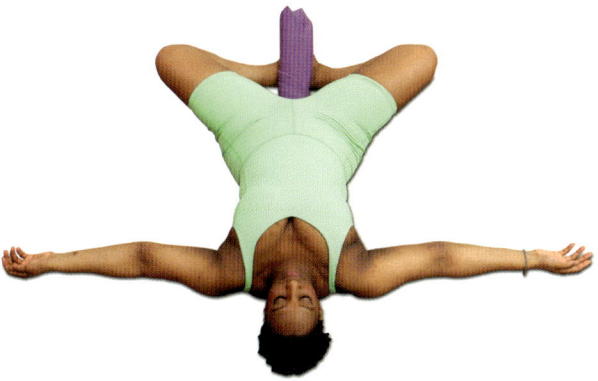

8.  Supta Baddha Koṇāsana with cone (page 79)

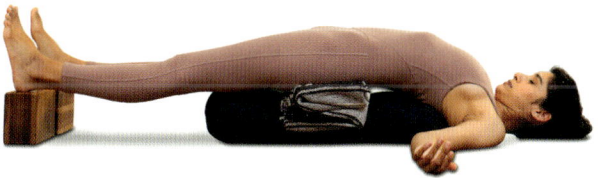

9.  Setubandha Sarvāṅgāsana (page 63)

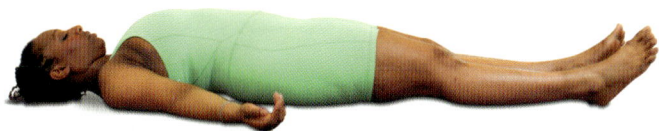

10.  Śavāsana (page 65)

# Week 3
## TONIFYING *the* PELVIC FLOOR

Once you've learned to release the muscles of the pelvic floor and have started to sensitize yourself to any areas of difficulty, we can begin the practice of engaging and strengthening the pelvic floor muscles. Many practitioners and newly postpartum people are quick to want things to "go back to normal," but you should take care to stay sensitive when learning how to engage and strengthen the pelvic floor. Strengthening happens slowly, with repeated practice, and may seem slow at first. Over time, however, you may begin to notice things like less heaviness or pressure in the pelvic region, a feeling of safety or containment, better endurance during other activities, and less pain in other nearby areas like the back, hips, or sacroiliac joint. Many students report feeling generally more balanced and stronger when doing regular daily activities like picking up a child or going for a walk.

In this sequence, you begin the art of learning how to engage and lift the pelvic floor. In physical therapy language, this is called a pelvic floor contraction or a Kegel. In yogic language we refer to this as *mūla bandha. Mula* refers to the perineal region located between the anus and the genitals, at the base of the pelvic floor. A *bandha* is a lock or grip in a particular region of the body; its purpose is to control the movement of breath and energy *(prāṇa)*. As pelvic floor dysfunction can occur when muscles are both overly tight or overly weak, you should use the āsanas in Weeks 1 to 3 to begin to understand your own pelvic floor "landscape" and to help determine whether practicing pelvic contraction is the right choice for you.

## PELVIC FLOOR CONTRACTIONS AND BANDHAS: WHAT'S THE DIFFERENCE?

### Pelvic Floor Contractions

If you've ever been advised to "do some Kegels," it's likely you've scratched your head, wondering *how* to perform what is more generally called a pelvic floor contraction. Here you'll find instructions to help you connect with, isolate, and coordinate the different layers of pelvic muscle. There is no one instruction that works for every body, so don't be concerned if you don't feel what is being described. It may take more practice or a different approach.

Pelvic contractions involve coordination of each of the muscular layers of the pelvic floor reviewed in chapter 1. Begin by orienting yourself to the inferior view of the pelvis, looking up from the bottom, and recall the shape of a diamond within the bony frame of the pelvis, made up of a front and back triangle (fig. 1.7). The front urogenital triangle surrounds the urethra and genitals, while the back anorectal triangle surrounds the anus, which leads to the rectum.

Bring your attention to the front triangle and specifically your urethra, the small opening where urine exits the body. To contract the muscles around the front triangle, imagine that you can draw your urethra back and in toward your body, like a telescoping action. Now try this movement in coordination with an exhale. Notice whether you can feel muscle activity around your front triangle and specifically around your urethra. Inhale and release this action completely before you practice it again.

Another technique that can help engage around the front triangle for those who have a clitoris, located just above the urethra, is to first imagine that you can nod your clitoris down slightly. Next try doing this action on an exhale. While you may not actually be able to nod your clitoris, you may develop an awareness and connection with the first and second layers of pelvic floor muscles. If you feel your abdomen harden or push out, or notice your buttock or inner groin muscles engage, reduce your effort and maintain focus around your front triangle.

Shift your focus toward your posterior or anorectal triangle, toward the muscles around your anus. First imagine drawing your anus up and in, like you're holding in gas. Do this action using an exhale and notice how it feels in your body. Are you able to distinguish between your buttock muscles and your anus? Breathe steadily, hold the contraction for a few seconds, then inhale and release it completely before you try again. Similarly to the front triangle, if you feel your abdomen harden or other muscles around the pelvis engage, particularly the buttock muscles, back off of your effort a bit.

The techniques described here have oriented you to how to find and isolate the muscles of your front and back pelvic triangles. You may find that for a period of time you have to focus more on activating one part of your pelvic floor or the other to address your specific needs. Once you can isolate the front and back of your pelvic floor, you can join these actions together for a more complete and full contraction of all three layers of pelvic floor muscle.

To do this, begin by lying on your back with knees bent and feet on the floor. Exhale as you engage the muscles of your pelvic floor, front and back, simultaneously. At first you may notice that you're holding your breath while you contract. With practice, eventually you will be able to breathe more steadily while holding your pelvic muscle contractions for a few rounds of breath. Inhale, release and rest the muscles of your pelvis completely before you try again. Also note that isolated pelvic contractions do not involve moving your pelvis in any direction; your pelvis should eventually be still as you contract and release these muscles.

## Mūla bandha

Performing a pelvic floor contraction and doing mūla bandha are very similar. The same muscles are involved, and the general instructions about how to initiate and visualize the movement are the same.

However, the term bandha means a lock or a grip and refers to a certain control of energy in the body. Imagine a great river that flows freely. It has one direction of movement. Now imagine placing a dam on the river. The water slows and becomes still, and you have controlled that great rushing river. Similarly, when we do mūla bandha, we are engaging the root lock, and the energy is no longer moving downward. In fact, we feel an uplifting of energy into the abdomen, up through the lower spine, and even into the chest and upper spine. This change in energy and our sensitivity to it is one way that doing mūla bandha may feel different from doing a pelvic floor contraction.

Other bandhas include *uḍḍīyāna bandha,* which translates as "flying up" and involves lifting and gripping the abdominal wall back and up after the exhalation. It is discussed in more detail in poses such as Mahā Mudrā (Week 3 pose 2) and in poses such as Utkaṭāsana and Ūrdhva Prasārita Pādāsana, presented in Week 5. Additionally, the chin lock, *jālandhara bandha,* is discussed in Mahā Mudrā.

It is important to note that not all practitioners may be ready to begin the actions of contracting the pelvic floor. If you have high tension in the pelvic floor, you should pay greater attention to the relaxing actions in the previous two sequences, though everyone can practice the prāṇāyāma in this sequence, which can have a deeply relaxing effect. When there is some progress in learning to relax the pelvic floor, you may begin with the contracting actions slowly and mildly, perhaps only giving half effort. Take care to see that the contraction is fully releasing. Additionally, people who are newly postpartum should wait until bleeding has completely stopped, and then proceed slowly with the āsanas in this sequence. Those who are menstruating should refrain from practicing bandhas and Mahā Mudrā (though one can make the shape of the pose without the bandhas), as well as the inversions, and instead should focus on the supported forward bends and prāṇāyāma.

# DEVELOPING A HOME PRACTICE

You may find yourself asking, "Which āsanas are best for me to practice? Do I keep practicing the previous poses or move on? How do I know I'm ready to go deeper?" Keep in mind that the sequences presented here are progressive and build on one other. You will see poses repeated week to week, which starts to give a sense of how you can build your practice. When you encounter poses that feel challenging, ask yourself whether you feel excited to try them and improve, or if perhaps you're not quite ready to take them on. Be patient and compassionate with yourself.

Here are some additional guidelines for developing your home practice.

If you only have limited time or are newly postpartum:

- Focus on the āsanas that feel meaningful, meaning those that aren't straining, give you energy, and help you connect with your pelvic floor.

- Focus on restorative āsanas (Week 1) until your energy returns.

- Just do inversions, once bleeding has fully stopped, as these will give you energy.

- Incorporate a few minutes of prāṇāyāma (Week 3).

If you have more time or are ready to go deeper:
Try putting Week 1 to 3 sequences together. For example,

- Standing poses followed by seated poses, then inversions, Śavāsana, and prāṇāyāma.

- Standing poses followed by supine poses, then inversions, Śavāsana, and prāṇāyāma.

- One or two poses from each family of poses ending with inversions, Śavāsana, and prāṇāyāma.

These are just a few examples, and many more variations of sequencing are possible. For more guidance on sequencing, consult with your local Certified Iyengar Yoga Teacher.

## Sequence of Āsanas: Week 3

### 1. Jānu Śīrṣāsana with Concave Spine (Head-to-Knee Pose)

Sit on the edge of one or two folded blankets with your legs stretched out in front. Bend your right knee out to the side, bringing your heel close to the pubic bone and the sole of your foot against your left inner thigh. Gently extend your right inner groin toward the head of your knee and move the knee down. If the knee doesn't come down to the floor, add the support of a blanket under your knee. If your groin is very tight and your knee is quite a bit higher than the hip, then additional height under the buttocks may be helpful as well.

Reach forward with your arms and take hold of the straight leg foot; if it is difficult to reach, place a belt around the ball of your foot. Hold onto the foot or belt with two straight arms, and as you extend your calf toward your heel, pull back to firm your shoulder blades into the back body (fig. 2.50). Draw your arms into the sockets as you lift and spread your chest, with shoulder blades and trapezius moving down your back. Lift the sides of your waist strongly, and move the back ribs in, without letting your abdomen push forward or hang. As you lift your chest, extend your neck and look upward, keeping your shoulders moving down, away from your ears. Stay and breathe for two to three breaths, and then return your head to neutral. Repeat on the other side.

**VARIATIONS**

TIGHT HAMSTRINGS OR BACK: Sit on more height, adding extra blankets until your lower spine is able to lift more easily.

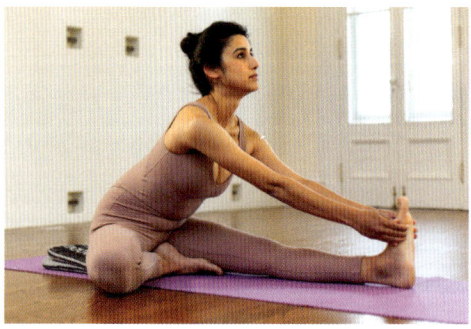

FIGURE 2.49. Jānu Śīrṣāsana

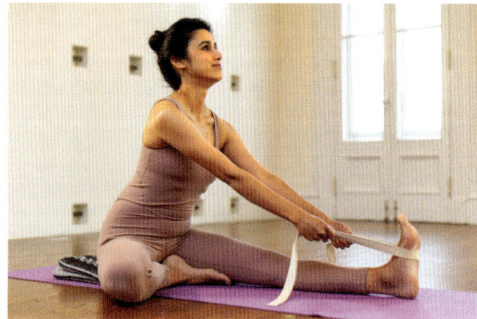

FIGURE 2.50. Holding with a belt

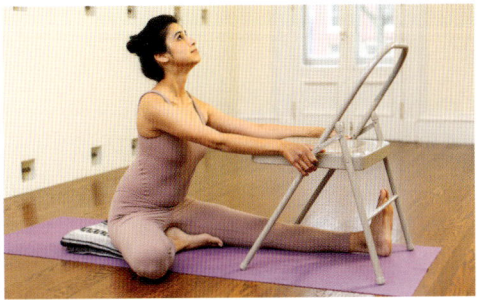

FIGURE 2.51. **Hands to a chair**

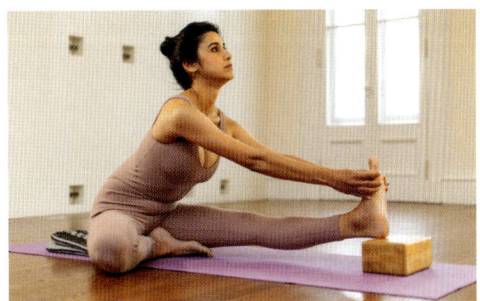

FIGURE 2.52. **Foot on a block**

ROUNDING IN THE CHEST AND SHOULDERS: Hold the sides of a chair instead of a strap to get a better lift in your chest (fig. 2.51). Alternately, sit facing the wall and walk your fingertips up the wall to help lift the spine up rather than letting it sink and cave in.

BETTER PELVIC AND ABDOMINAL TONING: If you have the mobility to do so, sit on the floor and place the heel of your straight leg up on a block set at its lowest height (fig. 2.52). The change in angle of the outstretched leg brings your pelvis slightly posterior, correcting an overly anteriorly rotated pelvis, which is common after pregnancy. In turn, it also helps to engage the pelvic floor and brings the abdominal muscles closer to the spine.

*Effects* *This forward bend, done in the concave stage, stretches and strengthens the spinal muscles, and begins the actions of tonifying the pelvic and abdominal organs as they are lifted and brought closer to the spine.*

## 2. Mahā Mudrā (The Great Seal)

Mahā Mudrā introduces the contraction of the pelvic floor muscles. *Maha* means "great" and *mudrā* means "seal," referring to sealing the body in a position to create a particular movement of energy. Traditionally, the pose is taught by inhaling and holding the breath while engaging the pelvic floor muscles in mūla bandha, the root lock. The abdominal muscles are also gripped and the organs are pulled upward, similar to uḍḍīyāna bandha (*uḍḍīyāna* means "flying up").

However, as many people have difficulty properly contracting and releasing the diaphragm and pelvic floor, it is taught here in a slightly untraditional manner—after the exhalation—so that the practitioner learns to synchronize the rhythm of the pelvic floor with the natural movement of the breath. The pelvic floor muscles are naturally contracted during the exhalation, so this method simply deepens this already occurring process. It also allows you to release more fully and naturally on the inhalation, which is an important action that we've described throughout this book. It may be helpful to visualize the movements of the respiratory diaphragm and the pelvic floor muscles, which are sometimes referred to as another diaphragm. They should move in sync with each other: lowering on the inhalation, and lifting on the exhalation (see "Diaphragms, Breathing, and Pressures" in chapter 1). Once you're comfortable with this natural rhythm, you can move on to learning the traditional pose in which *mūla bandha* is done after the inhalation. (This is not taught here; see B. K. S. Iyengar's *Light on Yoga*). Observe any differences you notice between these two approaches.

Set up as in Jānu Śīrṣāsana. Start with your right knee bent and your left leg straight. Holding onto the strap or the sides of a chair, press the root of the thigh of your extended leg down and raise the pubic bone up toward the breast bone. Now use the inhalation to lift your chest farther upward, and raise your head. On the exhalation, quietly lower your chin to meet your lifted chest; this is jālandhara bandha, the chin lock. In moving your chin down, watch that your chest doesn't cave in or sink down. At first, the chin may not come all the way to

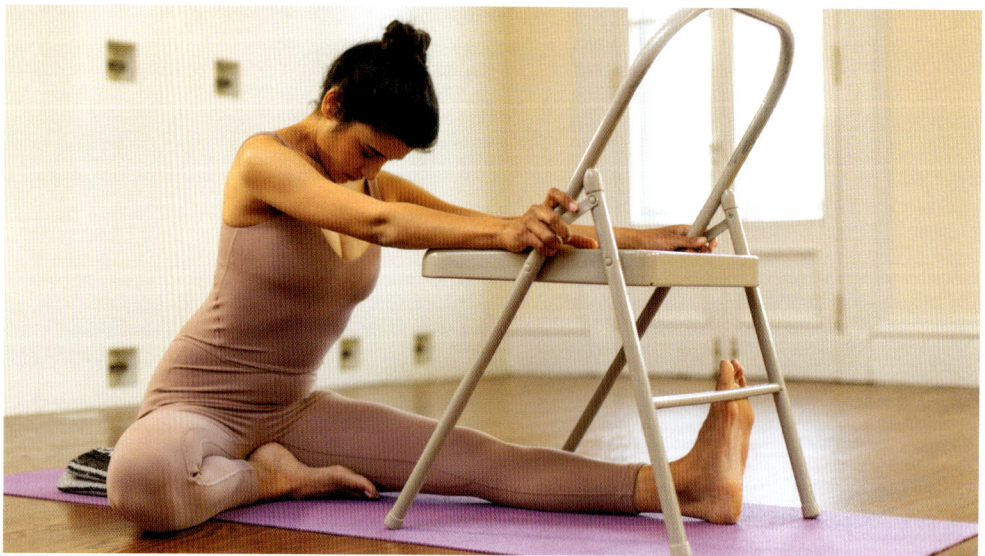

FIGURE 2.53. **Mahā Mudrā**

the chest. In this case, priority should be given to keeping the chest lifted. Stay for three or four breaths, keeping your spine lifted while maintaining quietness in your eyes, face, and throat. Observe the lifted energy of the spine from the base of your pelvis upward, while maintaining quietness in your head and brain. On an inhalation, bring your head up and change sides to repeat the pose.

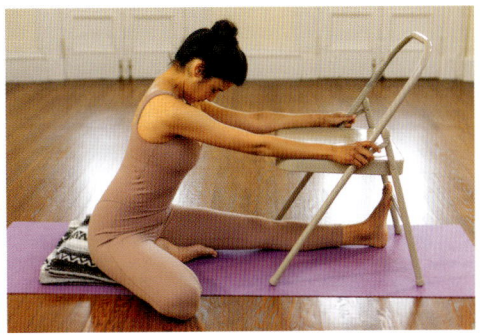

FIGURE 2.54.  **Side view.**

After you've become comfortable in this position, repeat on the first side, exhaling to bring your head down. Inhale slowly and gently, and soften and spread the respiratory and pelvic diaphragms (the pelvic floor muscles), keeping your chest wide and lifted. Then exhale slowly, and at the end of the exhalation, engage your pelvic floor by contracting and drawing upward. Draw your abdomen back toward your spine and upward into your chest. Hold for just a beat or two, maintaining the contraction, and then release your abdomen and pelvic floor on the inhalation. Repeat a few times, trying to synchronize the movement of your breath and the rhythm of the *bandhas*. This can be challenging at first as many people want to relax on the exhalation and engage on the inhalation. After repeating a few times, bring your head up and repeat on the other side.

Observe the difference in feeling between the inhalation and spreading versus the exhalation and engaging. Is one easier for you than the other? Are you able to contract only a little bit? Are you able to contract but not hold the contraction steadily? Are you able to fully release? Do the two sides of the pelvis feel the same or different? Asking yourself these questions and becoming attuned to your own tendencies and imbalances will give you greater sensitivity and awareness in your movements and your breath, inevitably allowing you better control and understanding.

## VARIATIONS

As in Jānu Śīrṣāsana, you can sit up on more height if your spine is not lifting well. You can also practice with a belt, a chair, or fingertips on a wall. If you have access to a rope wall, you can also hold the middle ropes.

**Effects** *This pose tonifies the pelvic floor muscles and organs, tones the diaphragm, and lifts the abdominal organs toward the spine. It also brings energy upward into the chest (prāṇa vāyu) and gently corrects the overly downward movement of apāna in the pelvis, which is predominant after pregnancy and childbirth.*

### 3. Jānu Śīrṣāsana with Head Supported

Place a chair in front of you, within arm's reach, and set up as in Jānu Śīrṣāsana, with the concave spine. Start with your right knee bent and your left leg extending straight underneath your chair seat. Keeping the chest lifted, fold forward from the hips, walking your hands up the side of the chair to further extend the sides of your trunk. Then maintain the extension of your spine, cross your forearms, and rest your arms and forehead on the seat of the chair. Observe the diaphragm and abdominal area again to ensure that these areas don't drop, which can put pressure downward on the pelvic floor organs. Your head should be well supported, not dropping down lower than the upper back, so that your neck can fully relax. Release your brain and the muscles of your face. Keep your spine lifted, and at the same time, relax any tension created from the previous poses. Focus on softening and spreading the pelvic floor with the inhalation. Stay two to three minutes, then repeat on the other side.

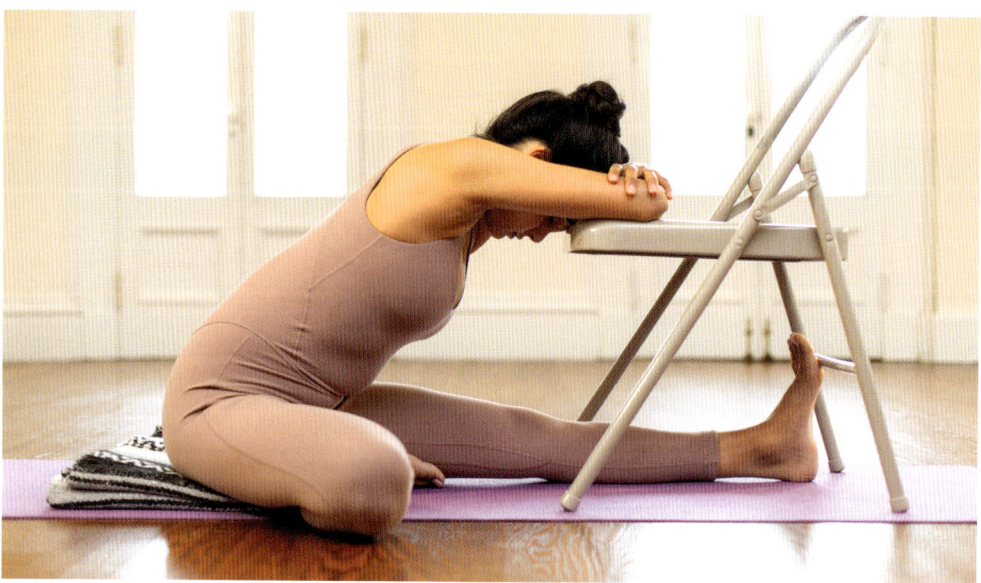

FIGURE 2.55. Jānu Śīrṣāsana, head on chair.

## VARIATIONS

STIFFNESS OR NEWLY POST-PARTUM: If your chest sinks in and your diaphragm and abdomen push back, use more height under your head and forearms (fig. 2.56). Those who are stiff or newly post-partum may need to add as much as a bolster on top of the chair seat.

*Effects* *This supported forward fold releases tension in the spinal muscles. It quiets the nervous system, relieving fatigue and anxiety.*

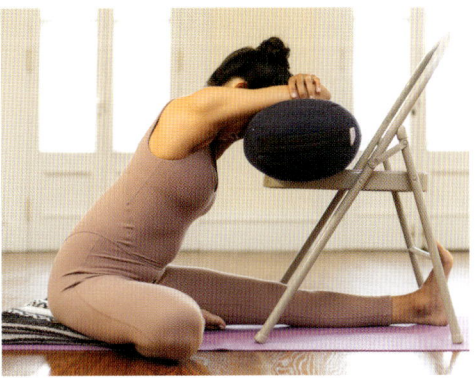

FIGURE 2.56.  **Head on a bolster**

### 4. Sālamba Sarvāṅgāsana

See fig. 2.57 and Week 2 pose 6 for instructions.

### 5. Ardha Hālāsana

See fig. 2.58 and Week 2 pose 7 for instructions.

### 6. Śavāsana (Supported)

Place a bolster vertically on your sticky mat, running parallel to the length of the mat. Fold a blanket and place it on the edge of the bolster (fig. 2.59). Sit a few inches in front of the bolster with your knees bent, your feet on the floor. Now lie back so that the bottom of your rib cage lines up and is supported by the edge of the bolster. If the bolster is too close to your buttocks and comes too much under your lower back, it can create

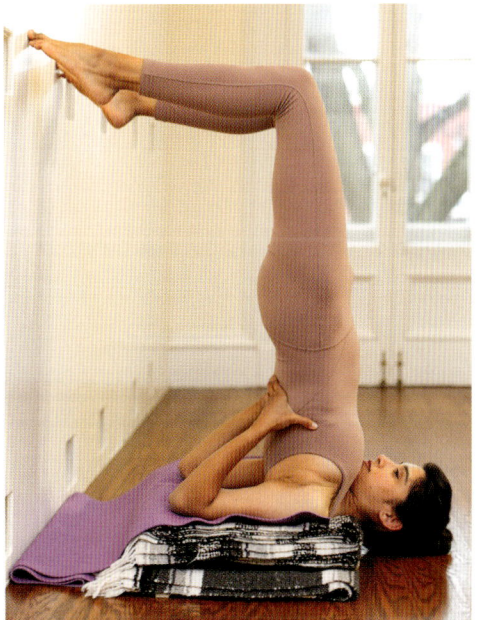

FIGURE 2.57.  **Sālamba Sarvāṅgāsana**

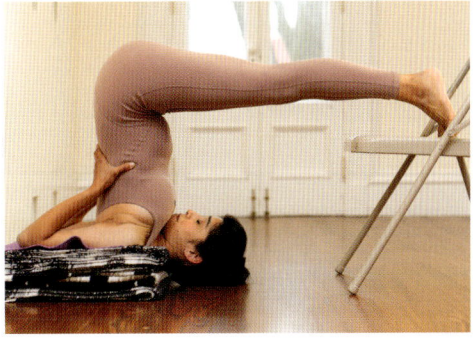

FIGURE 2.58.  **Ardha Hālāsana**

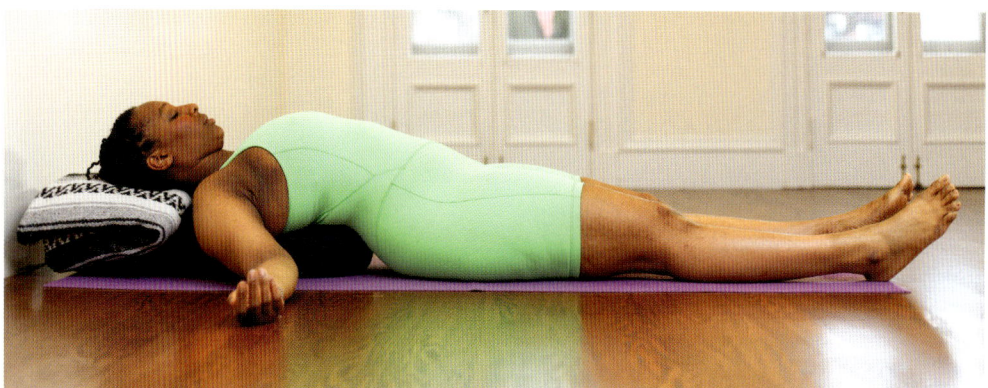

FIGURE 2.59.  Śavāsana supported on bolster

hardness in the abdomen. Move your buttocks away from the lumbar spine and move your tailbone in. Adjust the blanket so your head and neck are supported. Lengthen your shoulder blades down your back and lift and spread your chest.

Slowly extend your legs one at a time, observing that the pelvic region, abdomen, and chest all stay lifted and are not pulled down toward the legs. Relax your legs, letting your toes turn out, but keep your heels in line with your buttocks and not too wide. If the legs are too wide, you lose the containment of the pelvis and its organs. Relax your arms out to the sides with your palms facing up. Let go of any gripping in the body. Soften your abdomen, pelvic floor muscles, face, tongue, and eyes. Breathe softly and rhythmically. Observe any increased awareness of the movement of your pelvic diaphragm or any sensations that have been created.

## VARIATIONS

LUMBAR PAIN OR LUMBAR CURVE: You can place a folded blanket under your buttocks to lessen the curve in the lumbar spine. If back pain is acute, use one or two blankets folded the narrow way for your spine instead of the bolster.

TAILBONE: If there is no pain but it is difficult to bring your tailbone in, which is common in postpartum, you can use a rolled cone (as shown in Week 2, pose 8, and fig. 2.42) or belt the outer metatarsals of your feet, hips width apart.

*Effects* *In this supported Śavāsana, you can experience the stillness and quiet of the pose while effortlessly maintaining an uplifted and spreading chest. With your back ribs supported and your armpit chest broad, your breath aerates the trunk and brings freshness to the entire body. Supine prāṇāyāma can be done in this position.*

## 7. Ujjāyī Prāṇāyāma
## (Expansion of the Life Force or Conquering Breath)

### STAGE 1

Lie in supported Śavāsana. Begin to slow the breath, inhaling from the bottom of your chest to the top, and exhaling from the top to the bottom. Smooth out any disturbances in your breath, bringing evenness to all parts of the lungs. Create an even rhythm until the inhalation and exhalation are the same duration. The emphasis here should be on creating a rhythmic, sustainable, even breath, rather than a very deep breath. Keep your eyes, face, throat, and tongue quiet and keep your mind passive. Watch your breath with your mind, observing each movement, moment to moment. You can start with just two or three minutes and then build up to five to ten minutes.

*Effects* *This prāṇāyāma creates a soothing action for the lungs and diaphragm in preparation for deep breathing. It relaxes the sympathetic nervous system and creates steadiness of mind and spirit. Even a few minutes of practice can relieve fatigue and create a quiet mind.*

### STAGE 2

After several minutes in stage 1, you may proceed to stage 2, which is the lengthening of the exhalation. Take a normal breath in and then a slightly longer, slower, deeper exhalation, exhaling from the top of the chest to the bottom. Bring your mind deeply inside, tracing the movement of your breath all the way down. At the bottom of the exhalation, observe the slight pause before taking the next inhalation. Beginners should take normal breaths in between, checking to see that there is no pushing or overdoing in the breath. If you have more experience, you can repeat continuous cycles of Ujjāyī 2. While previously in this sequence there was emphasis on contracting the pelvic floor muscles with the exhalation, now there is no contraction. Here, the exhalation is used to create complete relaxation throughout the whole body. Rather than focusing on the particular region of the pelvic floor, try to bring your mind to the whole body and observe the effects of the exhalation throughout your body. Keep your face and mind passive as you continue to deepen your exhalations. Continue two or three minutes, gradually building up to five to ten minutes, and then return to normal breathing.

*Effects* *The emphasis on the long exhalation brings an even deeper, quieter relaxation for the entire nervous system and draws the mind inward. This can help ease anxiety, stress, insomnia, and fatigue.*

### 8. Bhrāmarī Prāṇāyāma (Bumblebee Breath)

Bhrāmarī means "bumblebee." This breath is done using a slow, smooth inhalation and then a sounded, humming exhalation, which resembles the sound of a bumble bee. To begin, lie in supported Śavāsana and exhale the breath completely. Now take a slow, smooth inhalation from the bottom to the top of the chest. On the exhalation, keep your lips closed and create a humming sound, feeling the vocal cords vibrate in the back of your throat. Different pitches can be used, but when first practicing, just use the pitch that feels most "normal" to you. At the end of the exhalation, inhale slowly and repeat, doing eight to ten repetitive cycles. After you have completed the cycles, rest with normal breathing, observing the effects of the vibration of the breath throughout your whole body, including your face, throat, chest, abdomen, and pelvic floor.

**Effects** *The humming vibration creates relaxation for the nervous system and may help you identify and release any unnecessary tension. Some practitioners may observe a connection between tension in the throat (udāna vāyu or the viśuddhī cakra) and tension in the pelvic floor (apāna vāyu or the mūlādhāra cakra), and that relaxing one area leads to relaxation in the other. Interestingly, if you look at pictures of the vocal cords, you will notice that they are shaped similarly to the vagina! The throat region is also sometimes referred to as another diaphragm, and the movements of the throat also work in rhythm with the respiratory and pelvic diaphragms.*

### Week 3 Full Sequence

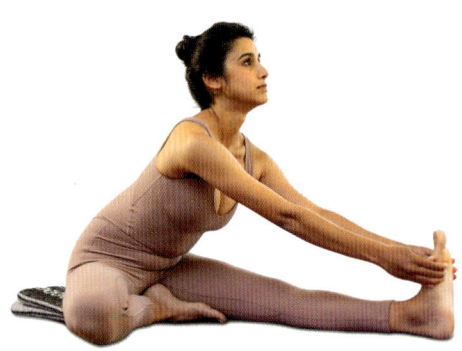

1.  Jānu Śīrṣāsana, concave spine (page 90)

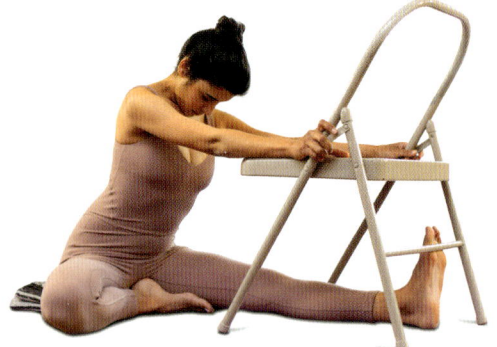

2.  Mahā Mudrā (page 91)

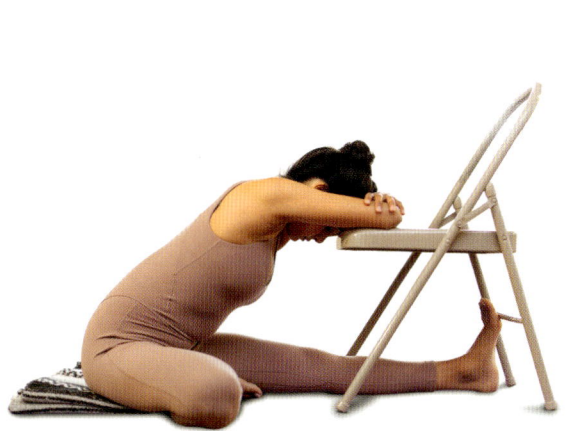

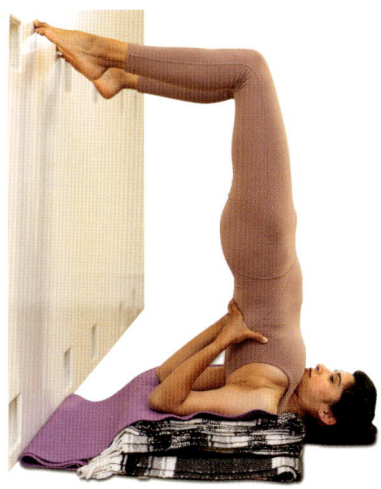

3.  Jānu Śīrṣāsana, head supported (page 94)

4.  Sālamba Sarvāṅgāsana
(page 75)

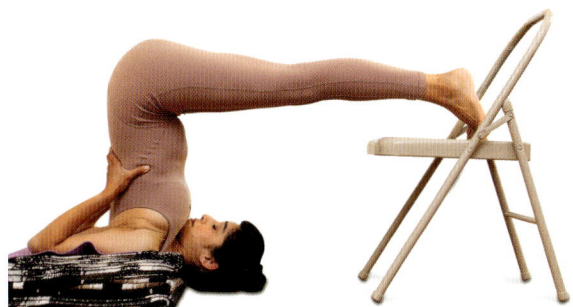

5.  Ardha Hālāsana (page 78)

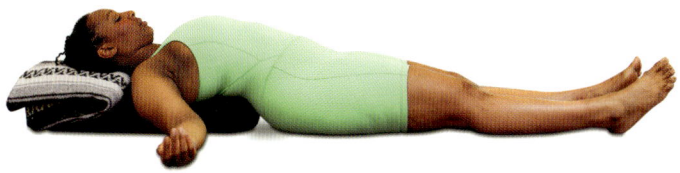

6–8.  Supported Śavāsana with Ujjāyī and Bhrāmarī Prāṇāyāma (pages 95–98)

# Week 4
# CONFIDENCE and STABILITY in STANDING and SEATED ĀSANAS

It is our hope that by now you've had the chance to experience the harmonious rhythms of the pelvic floor and your breath, and have increased both your awareness of this important region and also your ability to feel and control the muscles in the pelvic floor. As we progress to the next group of poses, we start to learn how to engage the pelvic floor while simultaneously taking the body through a wider variety of movements and actions. In this sequence, we begin a more energizing practice of standing and seated postures with the intention of teaching the body how to spread, engage, and lift the pelvic floor and organs in connection with the spine. We build on the strengthening actions in Week 3 as we add deeper legs actions and variations in the arms. Because the pelvic floor muscles are so closely connected to or associated with muscles of the hips, upper legs, lower back, and abdomen, there can be compensations that develop over time due to injury, weakness, trauma, or structural imbalance, whether in the pelvic floor muscles or in the surrounding muscles and joints.

As you move through the poses in this sequence, begin to notice other areas that might be feeling pain, tightness, restriction, or imbalance. How might these areas be connected to your pelvic floor? You may not know the answers right away—that's OK! Remember, be slow and patient on your healing journey, and try to notice connections, compensations, and imbalances with curiosity and openness. Keep building on these insights, and over time you can learn to balance the pelvic floor muscles in connection and coordination with all the other supporting muscles, bringing tremendous relief and healing.

We suggest that those who are newly postpartum should wait until about eight to ten weeks before beginning this sequence, and only then should begin with āsanas 1 through 8 until some stability and strength returns to the pelvis and pelvic floor.

## Sequence of Āsanas: Week 4

### 1. TĀḌĀSANA WITH A BLOCK

The instructions here as well as in the following few poses are similar to those in Week 2 but with a deeper focus on the pelvic floor and abdominal actions. Stand with your feet hips width apart and place a block at its narrowest width as high up toward the perineum as possible. Walk your feet slightly closer together so that the outer thighs grip in. Press the inner edges of your feet down as you lift from the inner arches to your inner knees, up toward the block. Try to lift the block up while keeping your legs straight and your knees firm. Roll the fronts of your thighs inward, and spread the backs of your thighs. Feel how this shifts the weight to your heels and helps open the backs of your legs. Lengthen the buttocks down toward the heels, away from the lumbar spine.

Move your tailbone in and forward toward the bottom of the pubis, while at the same time keeping the bottom of the pubis and the block moving back so that your thighs don't push forward. You can imagine the tip of your tailbone and the bottom of the pubis moving closer to each other. Notice whether you need one action more than the other: the thighs and block back, or the tailbone in. It takes some practice to develop this sensitivity, especially for postpartum people who may have a hard time bringing the tailbone in. Eventually you will feel both actions happening congruently. Once this alignment is achieved, lift from the top of the pubis to the navel as you lift the back ribs up, lifting and spreading your chest. Roll the outer corners of your shoulders back, stretch down through your fingertips, and soften your shoulders and neck. Keep your eyes neutral and your brain quiet and passive. Observe the feeling in your inner thighs, groins, pelvic floor, and lower abdomen. Soften your inner thighs, and try to grip the block more from your

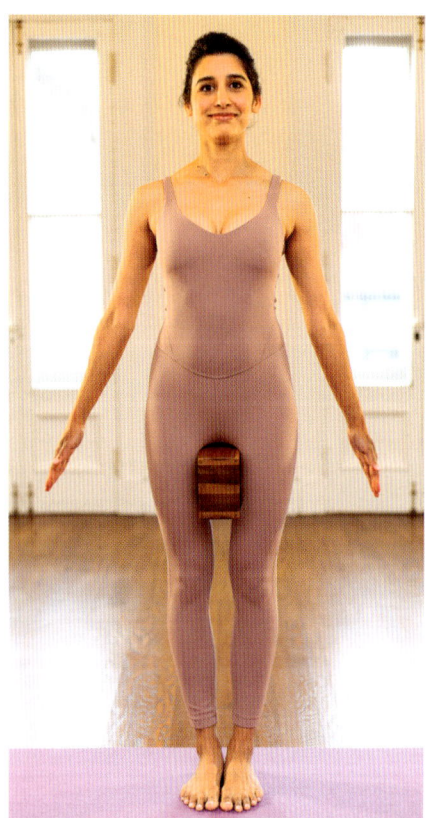

**FIGURE 2.60. Tāḍāsana with a block**

outer thighs, as you maintain the tailbone and pubic bone actions. Feel how these compacting actions in your hips help to lift the pelvic floor, creating space and stability for the pelvic organs.

Once the basic alignment of the pose is achieved, add a pelvic floor contraction on the exhalation. Make sure to relax your grip fully on the inhalation.

## EXPLORE

Some questions that might help you observe your pelvic floor in more subtlety in Tāḍāsana:

Am I able to bring my tailbone in and forward?

Can I feel the contraction of the pelvic floor muscles more clearly when my tailbone moves in?

Can I feel the pelvic floor against the block, and do I feel it lifting away from the block?

Where else in my body do I feel the lift: the abdominal organs, spine, chest?

**Effects** *This pose corrects misalignments in the pelvis and hips and helps stabilize the joints of the pelvis. It tonifies the organs and gives support and lift. Tāḍāsana with the work of the block simultaneously compacts the outer body but keeps the inner body spacious and lifted.*

### 2. Ūrdhva Hastāsana

The instructions here are similar to those in Week 2 but go deeper into the pelvic floor actions. Come into Tāḍāsana with the block as in pose 1. Keeping your legs firm and your spine lifted, stretch your arms overhead with your palms facing each other. Straighten your arms completely and keep your elbows firm, turning your upper arms so the outer arms (triceps) wrap in toward each other and entwine to the bone (external rotation). Soften your throat and jaw, and gently release your shoulders away from the ears.

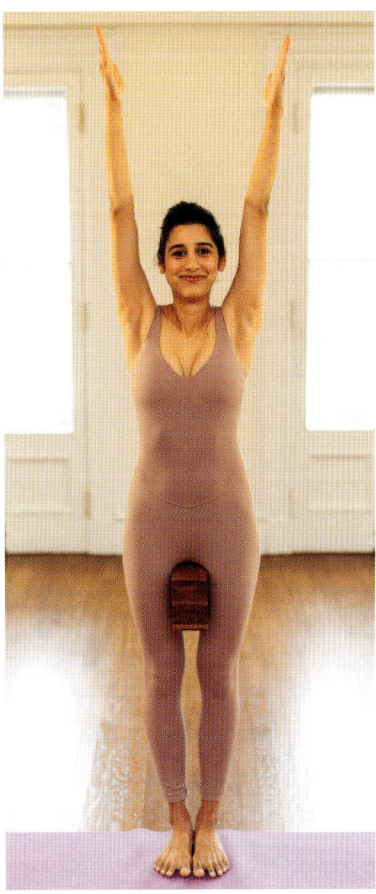

FIGURE 2.61. **Ūrdhva Hastāsana.**

Observe what happens to your legs, pelvis, and spine when your arms are raised. Were you able to keep the block in its place? Adjust your pelvis by pressing your thighs back and lifting from the top of the pubic bone to the navel. Now notice whether your front floating ribs are pushing forward. This can create unnecessary pressure on the abdominal and pelvic organs and is especially common for postpartum people. Soften the floating ribs back, spread the back ribs, and then lift up more from your back ribs. Now see if you can stretch your arms higher. Release your arms, coming back to Tāḍāsana. This āsana can be repeated a few times for better stability and alignment. Once ease comes to the shoulders and upper back, try engaging the pelvic floor muscles more strongly on the exhalation, releasing the grip fully on the inhalation.

### EXPLORE

Can you feel the lift of the pelvic floor aiding the stretch of your arms?

Can you connect the lift of the inner arches of your feet, inner legs, block, pelvic floor, spine, and arms?

### VARIATIONS

Tight shoulders or shoulder pain: Take the arms wider. You can also face a wall and walk your hands up the wall gradually.

*Effects As in Tāḍāsana, this pose gives stability in the pelvis and lift to the organs and spine. It helps to stretch the shoulder joints and opens the chest. You will feel more energy in your chest, and those with depression or sluggishness may benefit. Breastfeeding and chestfeeding individuals will also benefit from the opening of the chest and shoulders.*

### 3. Ūrdhva Baddhanguliyāsana

From Tāḍāsana with a block (pose 1), interlock your fingers, turn your palms inside out, and stretch your arms overhead. Firm your elbows and stretch your wrists, opening the skin of the palm toward the ceiling. Repeat the adjustments

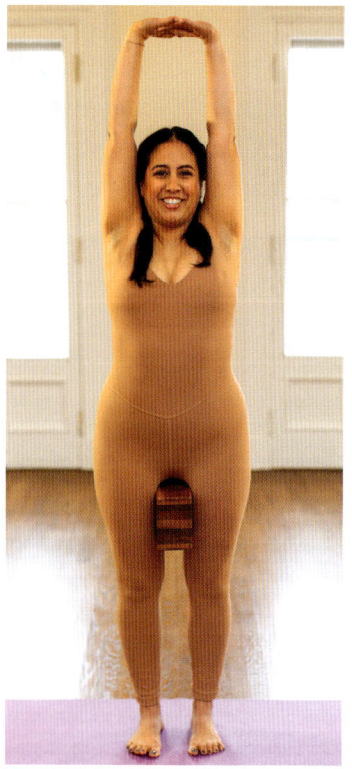

FIGURE 2.62. **Ūrdhva Baddhanguliyāsana**

as in Ūrdhva Hastāsana, keeping the block and inner thighs moving back and the tailbone moving in. Lift your abdomen and stretch the back ribs toward your wrists. Take two or three breaths here, then bring your arms down and repeat with the opposite interlock, with the other pinky finger on top. This can be repeated multiple times for better opening of the chest, shoulders, and wrists. Once ease comes to your shoulders and upper back, try engaging the pelvic floor muscles more strongly on the exhalation, releasing them fully on the inhalation.

**Effects** *This arm variation further lifts the torso, especially the back ribs. It opens the shoulder joints, stretches the wrists, and brings vitality and energy to the chest. This pose also helps breastfeeding and chestfeeding individuals with achiness and stiffness in the shoulders and wrists.*

### 4. Gomukhāsana Arms (Cow-Face Pose)

Place a belt over your right shoulder, and from Tāḍāsana, stretch your right arm overhead, bend your elbow, and place your hand on your back, holding the belt. Entwine the triceps muscles to the bone, bringing the upper arm and elbow in toward your ear. Stretch your left arm out to the side, turn your thumb to point downward, and bend your elbow, placing the back of your palm on your spine,

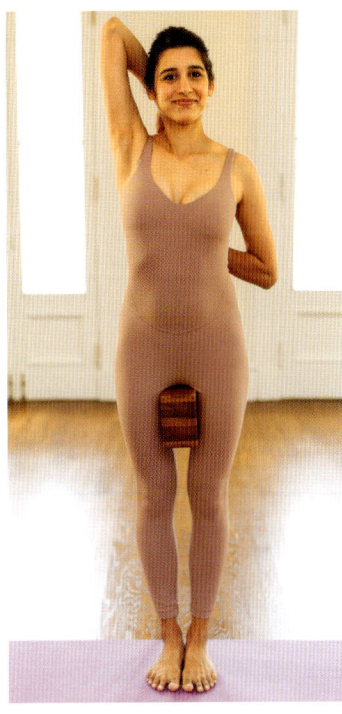

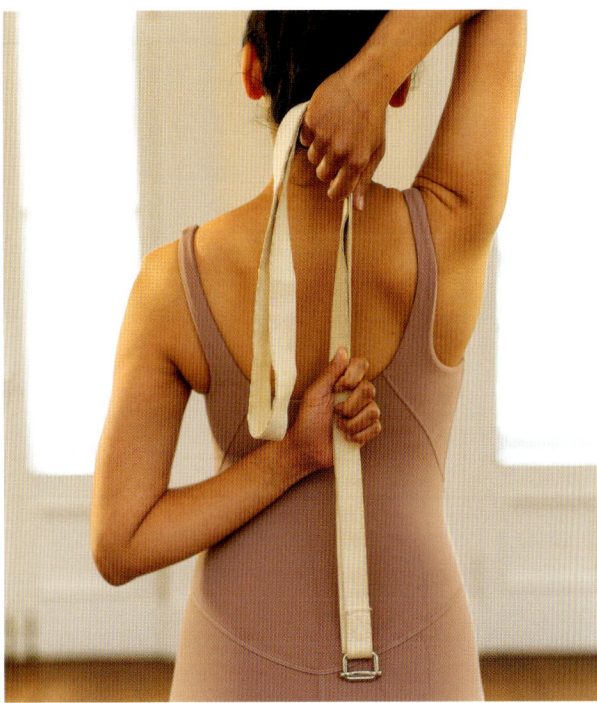

FIGURE 2.63. **Gomukhāsana**   FIGURE 2.64. **Back view, holding belt**

holding the belt. Lift and spread your chest and turn your left, lower arm from inside out, pressing your shoulder blades onto the back ribs.

At first, your hands will be far apart. The emphasis here should not be on getting your hands to touch; rather, establish the movement of your shoulder blades against the back ribs and the even lift of your chest. Because of tightness in the shoulders, practitioners often lose the lift of the back ribs in Gomukhāsana, causing the lower floating ribs to push out—this makes the abdomen hard and the pelvic organs drop. Therefore, take care to lift your abdomen and move the floating ribs back as you spread and lift the back ribs up. Stay for two or three breaths, then repeat on the other side.

**Effects** *This arm position further stretches the joints of the shoulders and arms, bringing increased mobility and circulation. It also helps breastfeeding and chestfeeding individuals with achiness and stiffness in the shoulders and wrists.*

### 5. Paśchima Namaskārāsana (Reverse Prayer Pose)

From Tāḍāsana, stretch your arms laterally to the side with your thumbs down and your palms facing back. Bend your elbows and bring your palms to touch behind you, turning the fingertips up. Turn the upper arms from inside out, roll the outer corners of your shoulders back, and press your shoulder blades onto the back ribs. Lengthen the backs of your arms toward your elbows, stretch from the elbows to the wrists, and now press both palms completely together. Once this is achieved, begin to move your hands farther up your spine. Maintain the lift of the back ribs and the spreading of your chest.

### VARIATIONS

Pain in shoulders or wrists: Grab hold of opposite elbows and forearms behind the back (Baddha Hastāsana). Alternatively, you can practice with

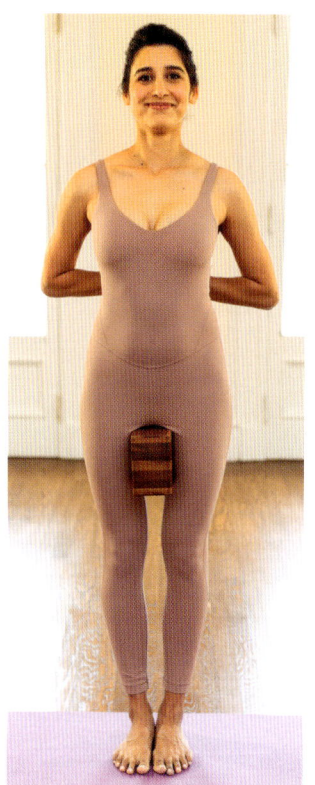

**FIGURE 2.65.** Paśchima Namaskārāsana.

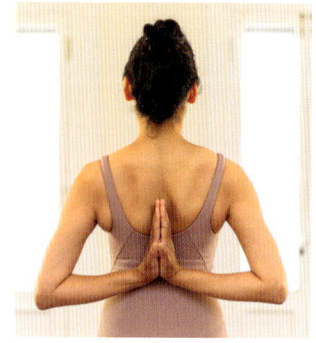

**FIGURE 2.66.** Back view.

your arms back and straight, fingers pointing down, with a belt tied around your wrists at shoulder width apart until more mobility is achieved.

**Effects** *This arm variation further stretches the joints of the shoulders and arms, and it highlights and corrects imbalances between the two shoulders. It opens the chest and armpits, bringing energy and vitality to the chest. It helps breastfeeding and chestfeeding individuals with achiness and stiffness in the shoulders and wrists.*

### 6. Vṛkṣāsana (Tree Pose)

Stand in Tāḍāsana with your back against the wall and no block. Bend your right knee out to the side, and bring your foot as high up your inner thigh as possible, touching your heel to the perineum. Press your foot into the thigh of your standing leg, and the thigh back into your foot. Your foot is now in the place that the block was previously in Tāḍāsana. Draw your outer thighs, buttocks, and hips in toward each other as you lift from the pelvic floor. Press the thigh of your standing leg back, keeping your heel heavy and leg firm, as you turn your right thigh from the inside out and gently move your knee back toward the wall, lengthening from the inner groin to the knee. Lift your spine and open your chest as you stretch your arms overhead.

Observe your back body against the wall and see whether both buttocks are even on the wall, with the buttocks moving down, away from the waist. At first, your buttocks may lift, and there will be a big gap between your lumbar spine and the wall; this may be especially pronounced for postpartum people or if the groins are tight. To correct this, bring your bent knee slightly forward, away

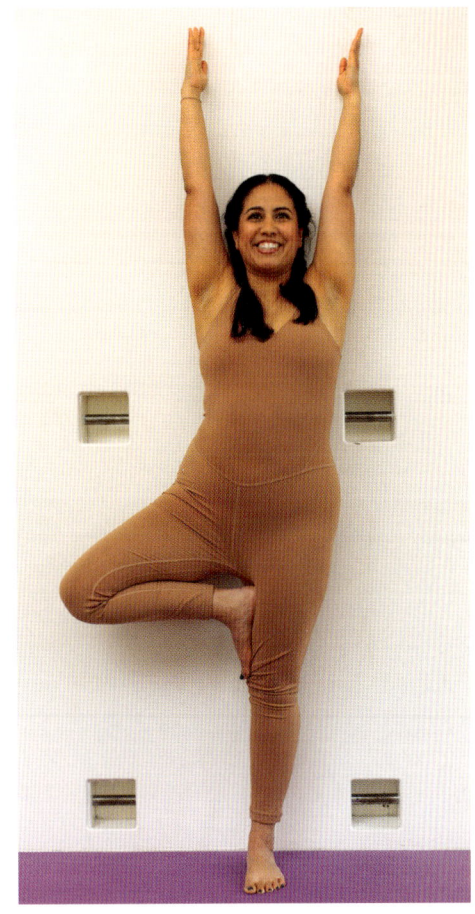

FIGURE 2.67. Vṛkṣāsana.

from the wall, lessening the stretch, and using your hands, push the buttock flesh down the wall toward your heels. Feel how this helps to lift the organic body up.

Once you are comfortable in the pose, you can begin to include small pelvic floor contractions on the exhalation, making sure to release completely on the inhalation. Observe how the pelvic floor contraction is aided by the actions of your legs, and how it helps the lift of the spine, chest, and arms. Stay two or three breaths, and then repeat on the other side.

**Effects** *This pose gently compacts the outer hips while spreading the lower abdomen. It brings lift and strength to the pelvic floor muscles.*

### 7. Utthita Trikoṇāsana (Extended Triangle Pose)

Place the short end of the sticky mat against a wall and angle a block, on its tallest height, at 45 degrees up the wall. Stand in Tāḍāsana in the center of the mat with your right side facing the wall. Step your legs wide apart, about four to four and a half feet, keeping your toes pointing forward. Turn your right leg out and place the ball of your foot up on the block. Line up the heel of your right foot with the center of the arch of your left foot. Lift from the inner arch to the inner knee to the inner thigh on your right leg. It can be helpful to keep your toes lifted away from the block to get this action. Turn the root of your right thigh out and draw the outer hips in toward each other. Press the outer edge of your left

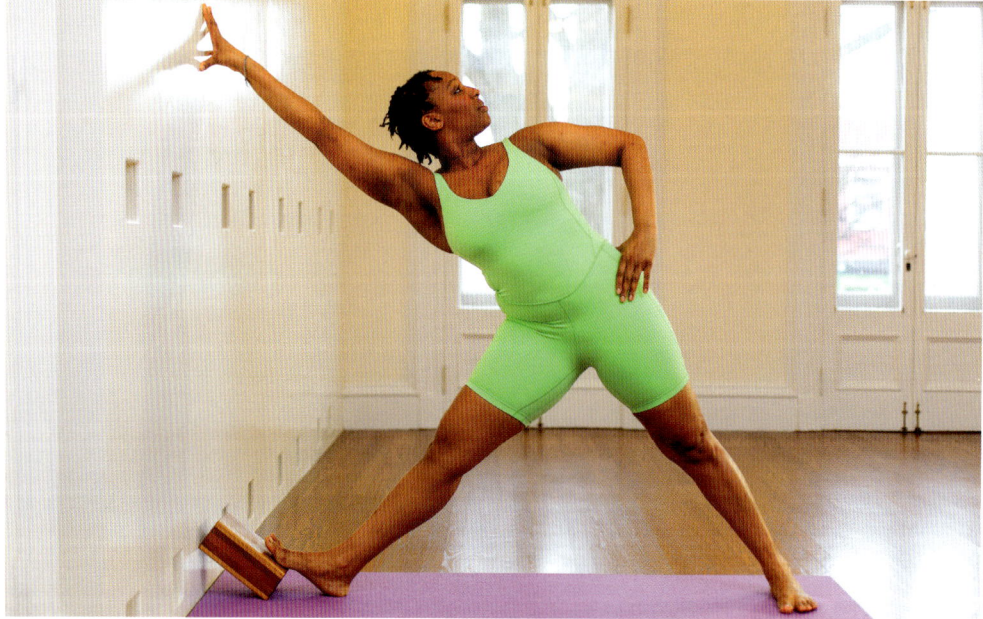

FIGURE 2.68. Utthita Trikoṇāsana, block angled at 45 degrees.

foot (the back foot) down, and press the root of your left thigh back. Bring your tailbone in and repeat the actions from Tāḍāsana, lifting the top of the pubis up to your navel and drawing your abdomen back. Now stretch your arms out wide, and keeping the extension of the right side of your trunk, reach your right arm toward the wall, walking your right fingers up the wall. Keep your left hand on your hip and roll your left shoulder back to open the left side of your chest. Your hips should shift to the left, with the root of your right thigh moving strongly away from the wall, but take care to maintain the grip of the outer thighs and hips. Lift the whole front of your body and turn your abdomen and chest toward the ceiling. The focus in this pose should be on the compacting and stabilizing actions of the hips rather than going for maximum stretch, as the pelvis may be unstable, especially for postpartum people. Stay for two or three breaths.

To come out, press into your back heel and stretch your back arm to come up. Turn your right foot in and carefully step (don't jump!) your legs together. Repeat on the opposite side.

## VARIATIONS

MORE STABILITY: Place the mat lengthwise against the wall near a corner, and practice with your back to the wall and your foot pressing against the block into the corner.

MORE ABDOMINAL LIFT: Do as above but face the wall. If going to your right, take your right hand down to your shin or to a block and take your left hand up, pressing it into the wall. Bend your top arm, and press with your fingers to help lift your abdomen toward your spine and turn it upward. This can also be done on a trestle or facing a half wall, ledge, counter, or banister, pressing your top hand down to lift your abdomen up.

GOING DEEPER: Place the block flat at its lowest height and move your heel all the way up on the block with the ball of your foot pressing against the wall (see the setup for Pārśvottānāsana, fig. 2.33, and Vīrabhadrāsana II, fig. 2.70). This deepens the action in the hip socket.

*Effects This standing pose energizes the legs and opens the groins while compacting the hips. The foot on the block brings the femur head deeply into the socket, correcting misalignment and instability, as well as aiding in some sacroiliac and hip pain. Some back pain may also be remedied. The better compacting of the hips gives lift to the pelvic floor, abdomen, and spine and ameliorates the downward movement of energy (apāna vāyu) after childbirth.*

## 8. Vīrabhadrāsana II (Warrior II Pose)

Set up as in Utthita Trikoṇāsana (pose 7), placing a tall block angled at 45 degrees up the wall. Step your feet wide apart and turn your right thigh out, stepping the ball of your right foot up the block. Make sure that your front heel is in line with the back arch of the foot. Lift your torso and bend your right knee to a right angle, keeping your knee pointing toward the wall and tracking over your toes. Maintain the firmness of your back outer foot pressing down into the mat, and keep your back thigh pressing back. You will feel the groins move in opposite directions. If you are recovering from childbirth, go slowly, as you may only need to bend the knee partway in the beginning. Keep your tailbone moving in and lift the entire front (anterior) spine up. The emphasis should be on keeping your torso upright rather than bending deeper into the groin. Stretch your arms to the sides, keeping the sides of your waist evenly lifted, and spread your top chest.

After attempting the pose a few times, you can begin to include small pelvic floor contractions on the exhalation, making sure to release completely on the inhalation. Feel how the contraction of the pelvic floor muscles aids the lift of the anterior spine and organs. Stay for a few breaths, then straighten your leg, turn your feet parallel, and step your legs together. Repeat on the other side.

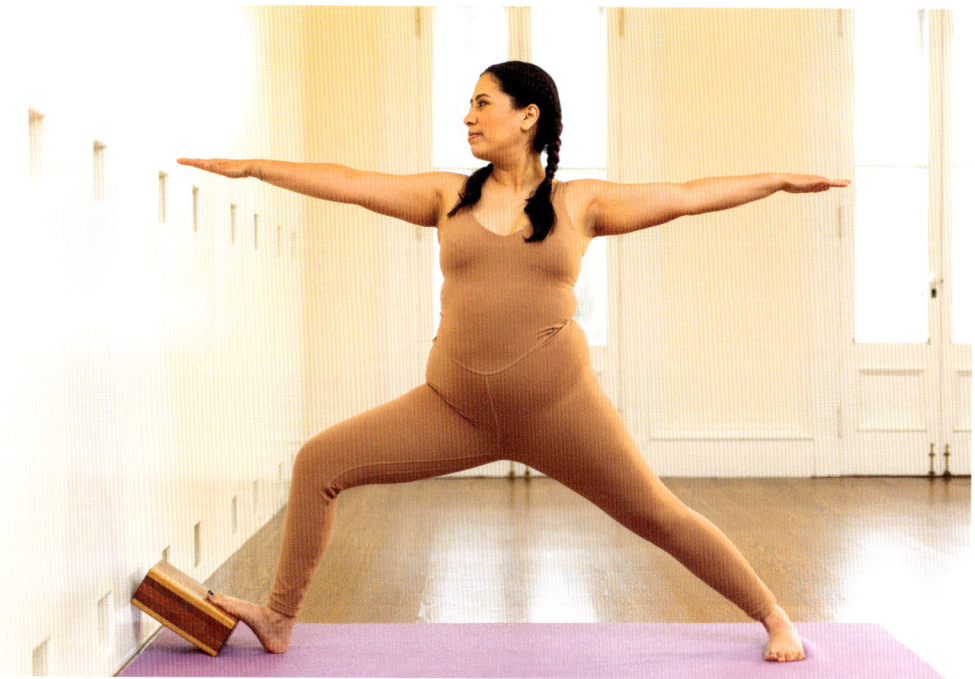

FIGURE 2.69. Vīrabhadrāsana II, block angled at 45 degrees.

## VARIATIONS

See variations for Utthita Trikoṇāsana, pose 7.

**Effects** *This pose opens the groins, making room for the tailbone to move in, and supports the lift of the pelvic organs. It brings vitality and circulation to the pelvis and helps correct imbalances and tightness in the hips.*

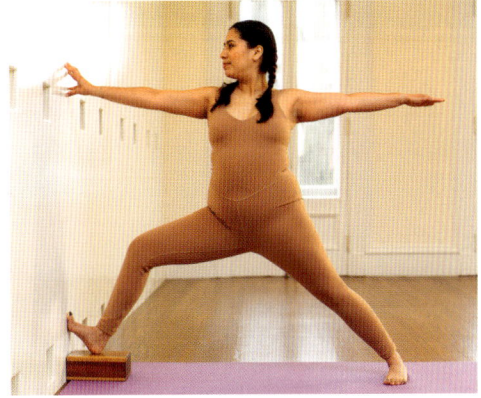

FIGURE 2.70. **Foot on a block at the wall**

### 9. ARDHA CHANDRĀSANA (HALF MOON POSE)

Place your mat lengthwise against a wall. Stand in Tāḍāsana with your back to the wall. Step your legs wide apart and turn your right leg out as you did for Utthita Trikoṇāsana (pose 7) and Vīrabhadrāsana II (pose 8). Keeping your back against the wall, reach your right hand down to your shin. Bend your right leg and step the back foot in, placing your right hand on a high block about a foot in front of your little toe. Put the weight into your hand, straighten your

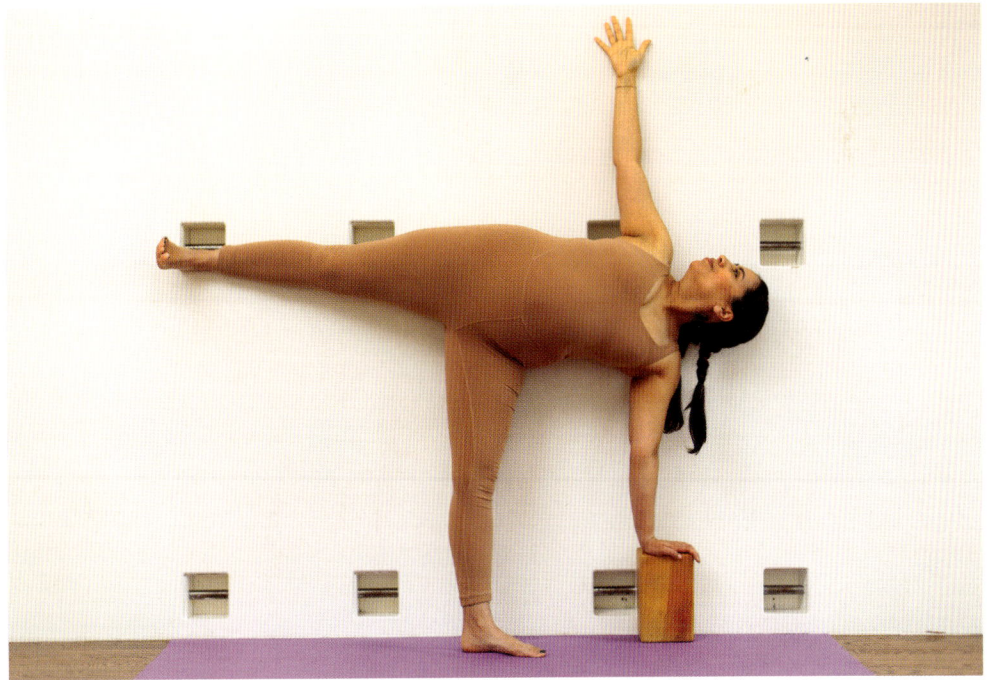

FIGURE 2.71. **Ardha Chandrāsana**

front leg, and raise your back leg up so that your left (back) foot comes in line with your hip (fig. 2.71). The foot of your standing leg will be a few inches away from the wall, the block right at the wall, and the heel of your back leg pressing against the wall if possible. Observe the standing leg: keep the inner arch of your foot lifting, firm your knee, and turn your thigh out so your knee points right over your toes. At first, you will feel your right buttock against the wall more than the left. Move your right buttock in, away

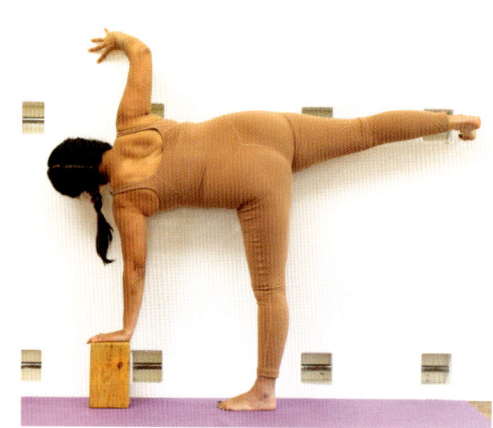

FIGURE 2.72. **Abdomen to the wall**

from the wall, and the root of your left thigh back, toward the wall, to "stack" the buttocks, opening the front of the pelvis upward. Lean back on the wall, bringing your lumbar spine closer to the wall, and move your buttocks away from your lumbar spine toward your heels. At first, this will be challenging work, as the abdomen and organs may have a tendency to fall away from the spine toward the floor. Work on turning your abdomen, ribs, and armpit chest toward the ceiling. Press your shoulder blades evenly onto the wall, stretching your arms in opposite directions. Stay for a few breaths, then bend your front knee and reach your back foot back and down to the floor. Come up and repeat on the other side.

### VARIATIONS

MORE ABDOMINAL SENSITIVITY AND LIFT: Practice with your abdomen facing the wall, using your top hand to press the wall, and turn your abdomen more (fig. 2.72). This can also be practiced against a countertop or high table for more support.

BACK PAIN: Stand with your back against a countertop or high table and rest your top foot on the counter. You can also use a high stool or trestle to support your raised leg.

*Effects This pose brings space, vitality, and circulation to the pelvis and abdomen, and introduces a mild twisting action to the organs to tonify them and bring them closer to the spine. It also brings lightness and joy to the whole body.*

## 10. JĀNU ŚĪRṢĀSANA (CONCAVE SPINE)

See fig. 2.73 and Week 3 pose 1. for instructions and variations.

## 11. JĀNU ŚĪRṢĀSANA (HEAD SUPPORTED)

See fig. 2.74 and Week 3 pose 3 for instructions and variations. After some mobility is attained, you can support your head at a lower height, such as on a bolster or folded blanket placed across the straight leg.

## 12. MAHĀ MUDRĀ

See fig. 2.75 and Week 3 pose 2 for instructions.

## 13. PAŚCHIMOTTĀNĀSANA WITH CONCAVE SPINE (INTENSE BACK-STRETCH POSE)

Sit on one or two folded blankets. Stretch your legs out straight with your legs together, reaching through the inner heels. Raise your arms up, lengthen the sides of your waist, and bend forward, catching the sides of your feet. Straighten your arms, draw your arms back into the sockets, and lift the sides of your waist strongly to bring the back ribs in. Lift from the pubis to the navel, navel to sternum. Spread your chest well. Stay for two to three breaths, release, and repeat, or proceed to the next pose. After some ease is gained in the pose, try introducing a pelvic floor contraction (mūla bandha) to increase the lift of the organs and the spine.

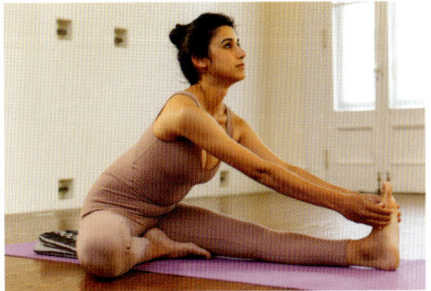

FIGURE 2.73. Jānu Śīrṣāsana, concave spine.

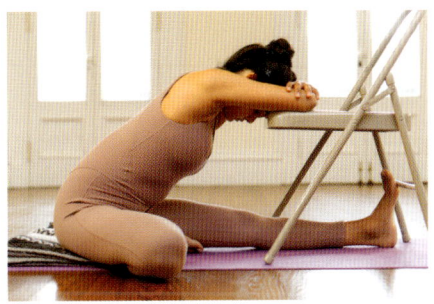

FIGURE 2.74. Jānu Śīrṣāsana, head supported.

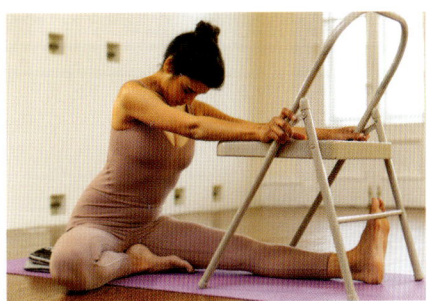

FIGURE 2.75. Mahā Mudrā.

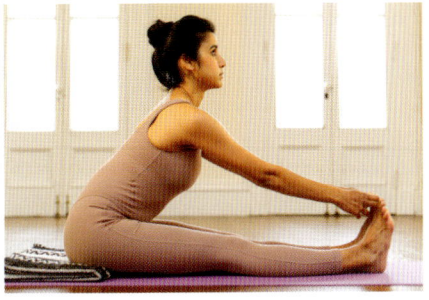

FIGURE 2.76. Paśchimottānāsana.

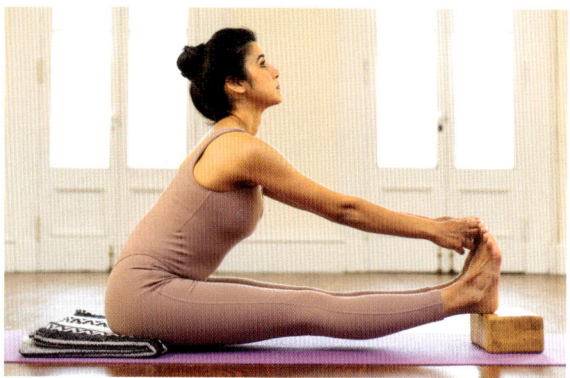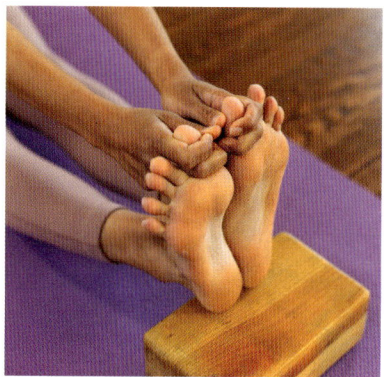

FIGURE 2.77. **Hands catching the big toes, feet on a block**

## VARIATIONS

TIGHT HAMSTRINGS: Sit on a bolster. Use a belt or chair for your hands as in Jānu Śīrṣāsana (pose 10).

NEWLY POSTPARTUM INDIVIDUALS: If it feels uncomfortable to bring your legs together, keep them slightly apart.

GOING DEEPER: Place your heels on a block to help better tone the organs toward the spine (fig. 2.77).

***Effects*** *This pose tones the back muscles as well as brings mobility to the hamstrings and freedom in the forward movement of the pelvis. It also tonifies the organs as they are lifted upward and toward the spine.*

## 14. Paśchimottānāsana (Full Pose)

Once lift and mobility are achieved in the concave stage, begin to bring your torso toward your legs, keeping your spine lengthening. The movement should come from the backs of your thighs to your buttocks, buttocks toward the lumbar spine, rather than rounding the spine. Spread the elbows wide and keep them slightly lifted in order to keep the armpits wide and the chest broad. Move the sides of your waist forward toward your armpits. Go slowly and observe when you begin to lose length in the front body. Postpartum individuals especially need to go slowly. If the back rounds too much, the organs will be pushed backward and downward, creating pressure on the uterus, bladder, and rectum. The emphasis should be on maintaining length in your spine rather than bringing your head down. The head can be supported by a bolster (fig. 2.79), blankets, or a chair, according to your capacity.

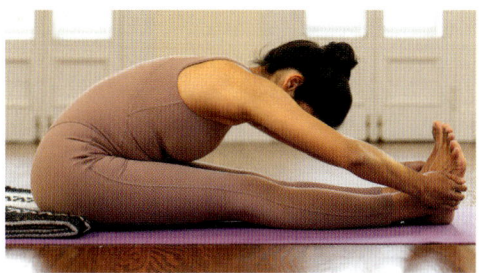

FIGURE 2.78. **Head toward the legs**

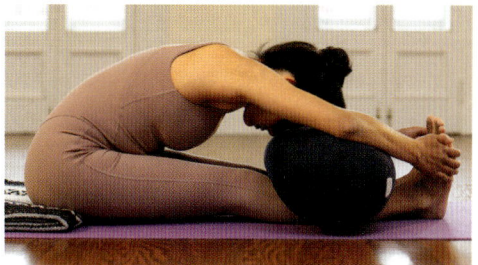

FIGURE 2.79. **Head on a bolster**

## VARIATIONS

TIGHT HAMSTRINGS: Sit on a bolster. Use a belt or chair for your hands as in Jānu Śīrṣāsana (pose 10).

**Effects** *This forward bend further tonifies the organs, bringing a gentle compactness and massaging action to them. The legs, pelvis, and spinal muscles are stretched farther. The head being supported brings quietness and calmness to the brain and relieves fatigue and anxiety.*

### 15. BHARADVĀJĀSANA I WITH A CHAIR (SAGE BHARADVĀJA'S TWIST POSE)

Sit sideways in a chair, starting with your right hip closest to the back of the chair. See that your feet and knees are forming a right angle. Press your outer hips in to create compactness as you lift your arms and lengthen the sides of your body upward. Twist toward the backrest of the chair and hold the outer rounded corners of the chair, keeping your torso lifted. Bend your elbows out to the sides and spread your shoulder blades laterally, bringing them down and in to open your chest as you turn. Keeping your hips and legs firm, turn your waist, chest, and armpits to the right. Take two or three breaths, and then release and repeat on the other side.

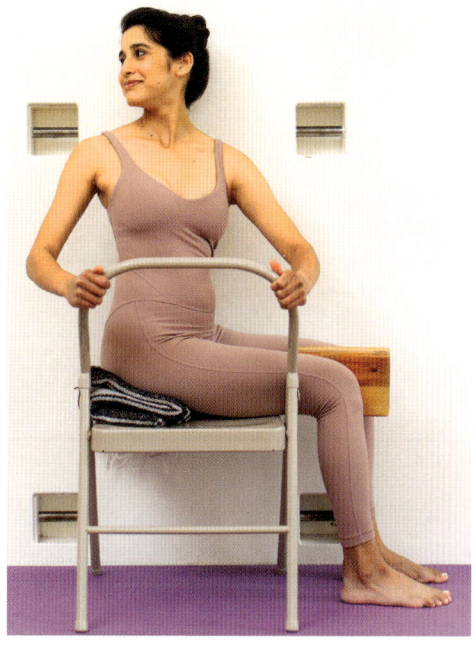

FIGURE 2.80. **Bharadvājāsana**

## VARIATIONS

Practice placing a block between your knees or thighs and hug your outer hips in. Can you feel similar effects as you did in Tāḍāsana with the block? This variation can help improve stability and compactness in the hips, lift the pelvic organs, and give better relief to the lower back.

**Effects** *This twist brings a wringing effect to the organs and spine, improving circulation and digestion. It relieves backache, especially after forward bending.*

### 16. SĀLAMBA SARVĀṄGĀSANA

See fig. 2.81 and Week 2 pose 6 (stage 3) for instructions and variations.

### 17. ARDHA HĀLĀSANA

See fig. 2.82 and Week 2 pose 7 for instructions and variations.

### 18. ŚAVĀSANA

See fig. 2.83 and Week 1 pose 9 for instructions.

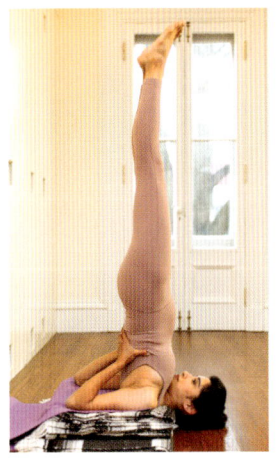

FIGURE 2.81. **Sālamba Sarvāṅgāsana**

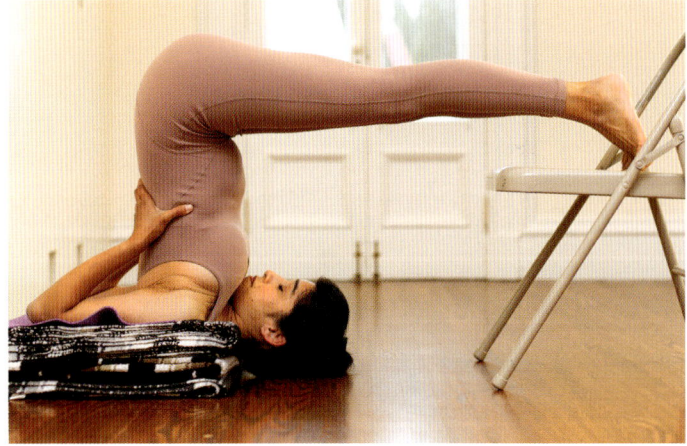

FIGURE 2.82. **Ardha Hālāsana**

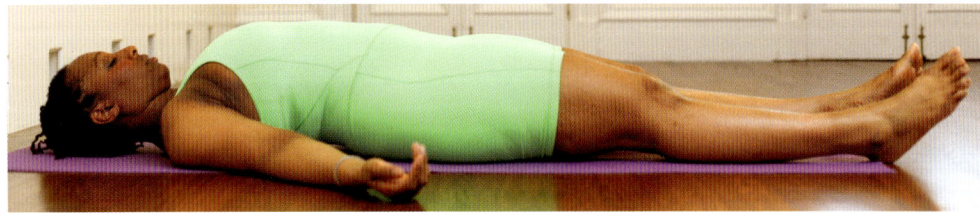

FIGURE 2.83. **Śavāsana**

## WEEK 4 FULL SEQUENCE

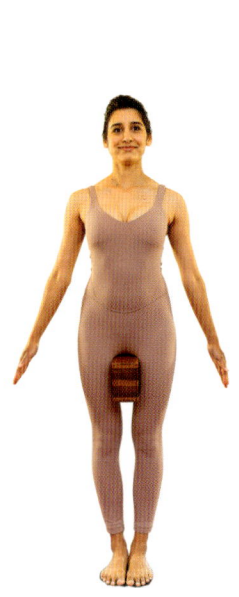 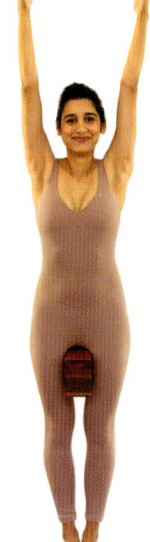 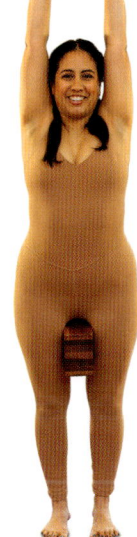 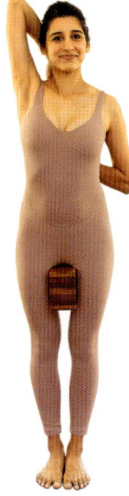 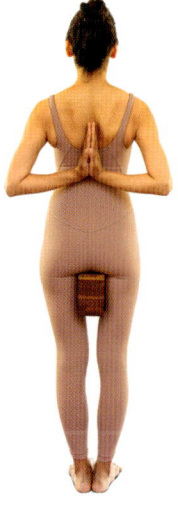

1. Tāḍāsana with a block (page 102)

2. Ūrdhva Hastāsana (page 103)

3. Ūrdhva Baddhanguliyāsana (page 104)

4. Gomukhāsana arms (page 105)

5. Paśchima Namaskārāsana (page 106)

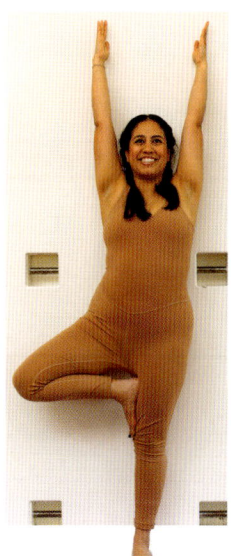 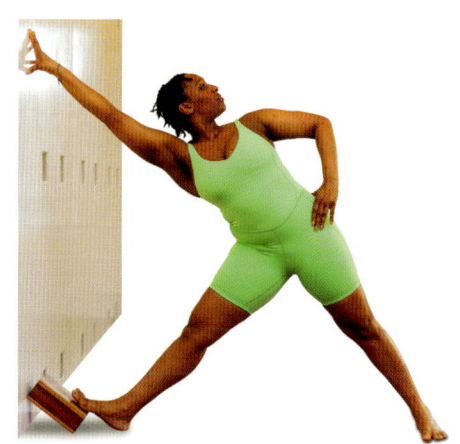

6. Vṛkṣāsana (page 107)      7. Utthita Trikoṇāsana (page 108)

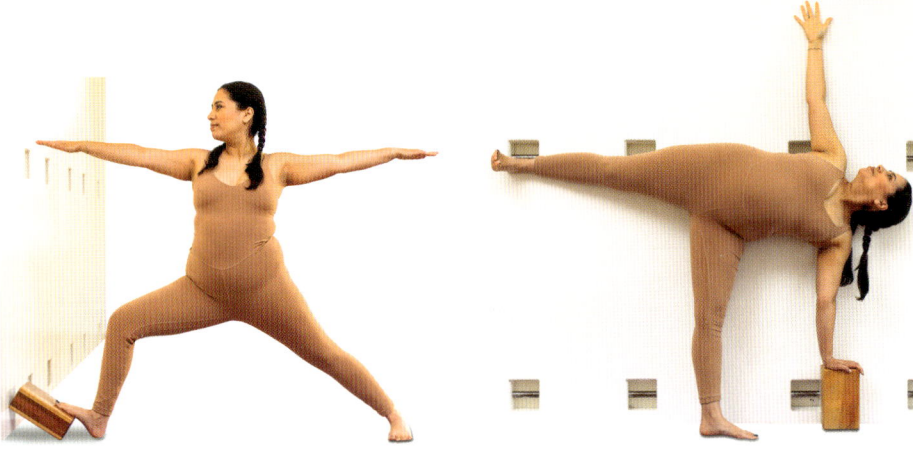

8. Vīrabhadrāsana II (page 110)

9. Ardha Chandrāsana (page 111)

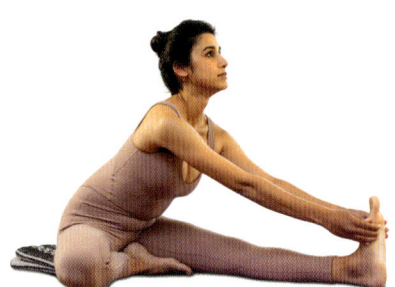

10. Jānu Śīrṣāsana, concave spine (page 90)

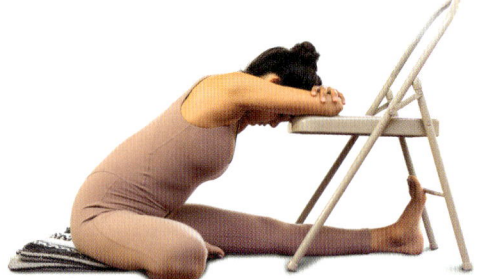

11. Jānu Śīrṣāsana, head supported (page 94)

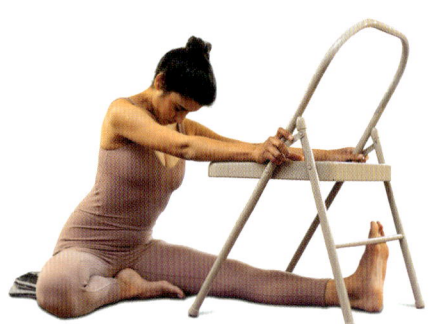

12. Mahā Mudrā (page 91)

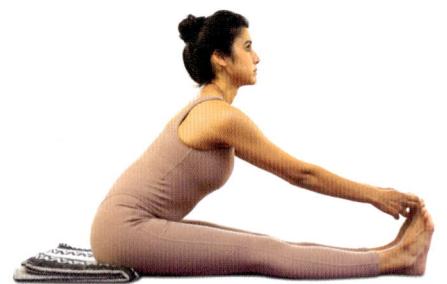

13. Paśchimottānāsana, concave spine (page 113)

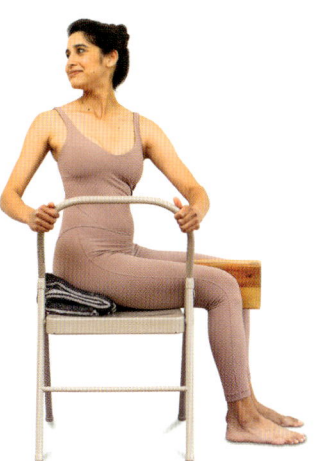

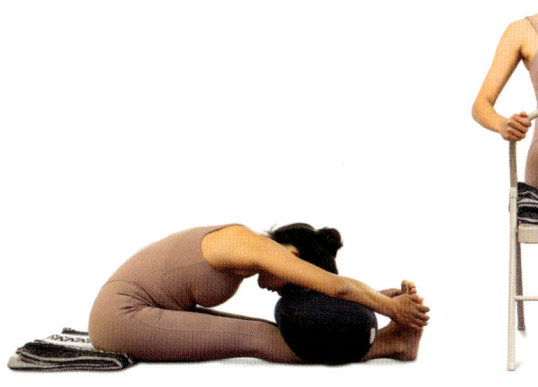

14. Paśchimottānāsana, forward bend with head support (page 114)

15. Bharadvājāsana (page 115)

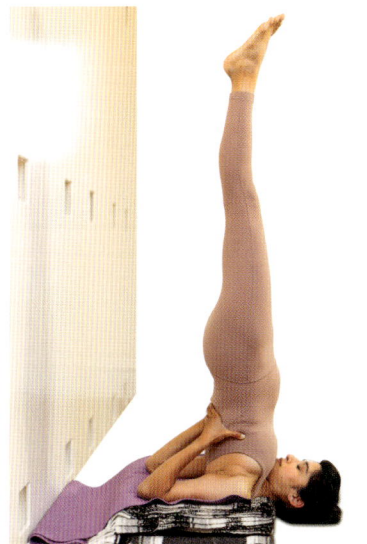

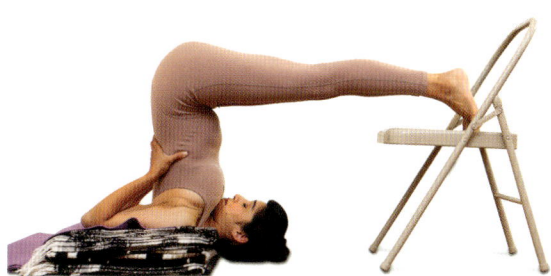

16. Sālamba Sarvāṅgāsana (page 77)

17. Ardha Hālāsana (page 78)

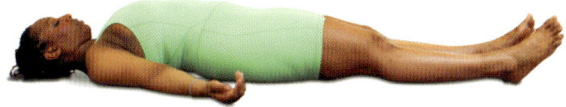

18. Śavāsana (page 65)

# Week 5
# FROM the GROUND to the CORE

When we think of doing "core" work, most people have an image in their mind of strong six-pack abs and lots of sit-ups. However, treating the core as one set of muscles is very limited and isolated, as it is in fact made up of several groups of muscles that overlap and interdigitate, creating a web of supportive actions and functions. Furthermore, in yoga, when we reference the core, we are also referring to the organs that are housed in the abdominal cavity as well the energies *(vāyus)* that move there.

Building on the actions of the previous sequence, this sequence introduces deeper work in standing poses as well as beginning explorations into abdominal work. Building from the ground up, we begin to understand the connections between the legs, pelvis, and abdominal cavity and how to remedy the overly downward movement of the pelvic contents after pregnancy and childbirth. It may be helpful to begin thinking of your core as a multilayered container, and though you may not have an exact picture, start to observe what is happening inside that container. Is there pressure? Do you feel pain or tenderness? Are you able to connect with the front, sides, back, and top and bottom of your container? These kinds of inquiries will start to deepen your connection to your core.

## THE CORE AS A CONTAINER

### The Anatomical Core

As described in chapter 1, the anatomical "core" refers to the muscular container that encompasses the lower thoracic and entire lumbar spine, the three layers of pelvic floor muscles, your respiratory diaphragm, deep spinal muscles, and your transverse abdominal muscles. These muscles form a circumferential container between your front and back, with your respiratory diaphragm at the top and your pelvic floor muscles at the bottom, creating a stable vessel that, when in balance, aids in healthy and efficient movement and supports our necessary internal pressures.

## The Yogic Core and the Vāyus

With an understanding of the musculature that makes up the core, we can more easily begin to picture this region as the home for the pelvic organs. As in any home, our container needs to be sturdy and firm, but we also need room inside to move around with ease. Too much tension or forceful action can disrupt the proper placement and functioning of the organs and cause instances of unwanted pressure on the abdominal and pelvic cavities. As we breathe, the top and the bottom of our container should move, allowing pressures inside our container to change and shift. In yogic language we call these *vāyu* (literally "wind" or "air"). The *samāna vāyu* (middle wind) moves in the region of the abdomen and collects, absorbs, and metabolizes energy brought into the body. It controls processes like digestion. The *apāna vāyu* (downward wind) moves in the region of the pelvis and controls elimination and childbirth. The *prāṇa vāyu* moves in the region of the chest, absorbing breath. Additionally the *udāna vāyu*, at the region of the throat, controls intake of food and air, and the *vyāna vāyu* travels throughout the body, distributing breath and nutrients from food. When these vāyus are in balance, we feel energized, balanced, and have ease and efficiency in the function of our organs. With pelvic floor health and postpartum recovery, we are particularly concerned with the balance between the prāṇa vāyu, samāna vāyu, and apāna vāyu. Pregnancy and childbirth create a lot of downward movement, and apāna can become out of balance.

As discussed previously, our breathing patterns can greatly affect the movements of the vāyus and the corresponding intra-abdominal and pelvic pressures (see "Diaphragms, Breathing, and Pressures" in chapter 1 and the sequences for Weeks 1 to 3). Being able to sense and feel these vāyus can greatly aid your work in the āsanas as you become able to adjust more intelligently, becoming more sensitive to the changes within.

Stability and endurance in the previous sequences should be established before moving on to this sequence. Postpartum individuals especially need to take care not to rush into doing abdominal work vigorously, especially when postpartum symptoms are present. You should proceed slowly with the correct understanding of the actions in each pose. Several poses are carried over from the previous sequence, and once you feel comfortable and familiar with the āsanas in Weeks 4 and 5, they can be combined, taking your endurance into account and if time allows. For example, you could start with Tāḍāsana and arm variations from Week 4 and then proceed with the beginning of Week 5. Seated poses could be practiced between Ardha Chandrāsana and Ūrdhva Prasārita Pādāsana. Those who are menstruating should avoid Ūrdhva Prasārita Pādāsana, Supta Pādāṇguṣṭhāsana I and all inversions.

## Sequence of Āsanas: Week 5

### 1. ADHO MUKHA ŚVĀNĀSANA WITH HANDS AT THE WALL (DOWNWARD-FACING DOG POSE)

Start on your hands and knees facing a wall. Place a block at its narrowest width as high up between your thighs as possible so the block touches your perineum. Turn your palms out 90 degrees on the mat so that your thumb and index finger meet the wall, keeping your fingers spread, hands shoulder width apart. Press your palms and lift your knees and hips up, straightening your legs. Press from your hands to your hips, straightening your arms and pulling the

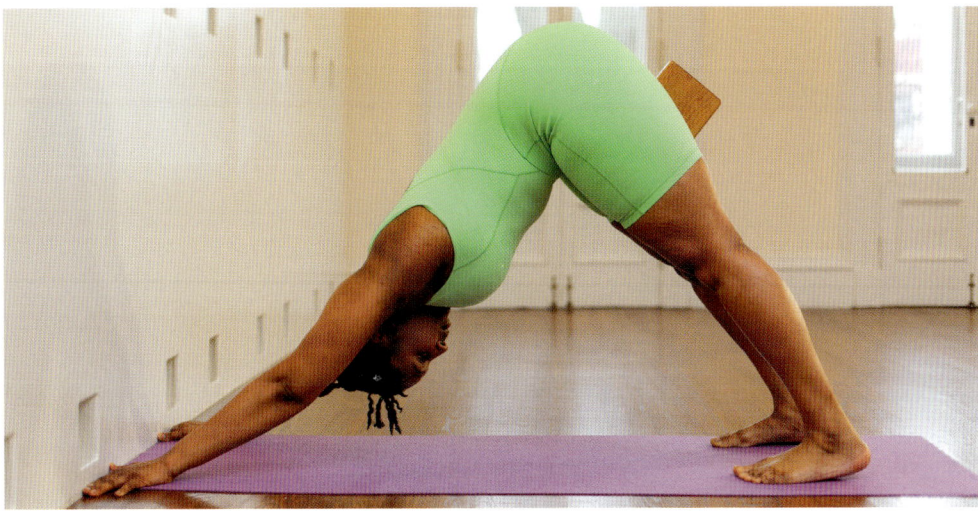

FIGURE 2.84. **Adho Mukha Śvānāsana, hands at the wall.**

sides of your torso strongly up toward the hips. Keep your upper arms turning from inside out and press your shoulder blades into the back ribs, moving your upper back away from the wall. Raise your heels and lift from the backs of your thighs toward the buttocks, lifting the block as high up as possible. Move your inner groins back to move the block back, but keep your outer thighs compact and moving back. Keep the backs of your thighs spreading to create space in the pelvic floor, and stretch from the crown of your head to your perineum. Stay for one to three breaths. Then bend the knees, come down, and rest.

The inverted action in the pelvis changes the organs' relationship to gravity. Observe the following:

Can I feel the double action of spreading the back of my thighs and pelvic floor as well as bringing my outer hips back and compacting my hips?

Do I need one of these actions more than the other in my body?

What is the feeling in my pelvic floor and abdomen: lift, space, and so on?

**Effects** *This pose inverts the pelvis, bringing relief to pelvic organ pressure or prolapse. It energizes the shoulders and spine and tonifies the organs toward the spine. Having the hands at the wall helps to further open the shoulders.*

### 2. Adho Mukha Śvānāsana with Heels at the Wall

Repeat the instructions for Adho Mukha Śvānāsana (pose 1), but place the backs of your heels at the wall and your hands facing forward.

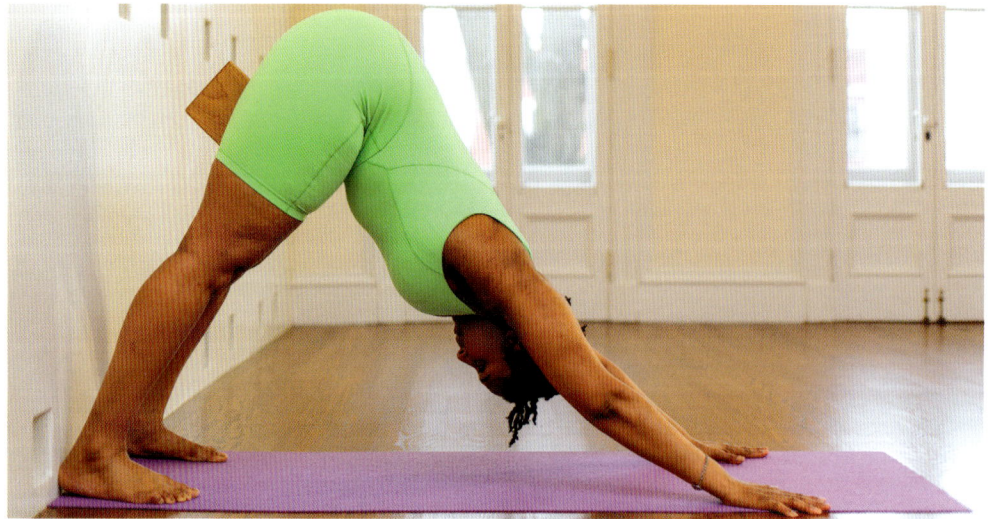

FIGURE 2.85. **Adho Mukha Śvānāsana, heels at the wall**

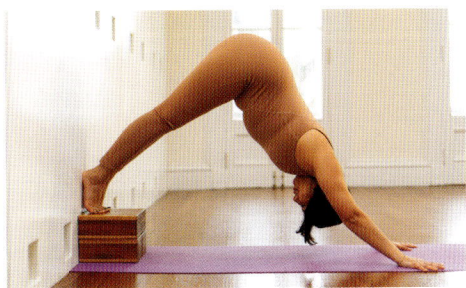

FIGURE 2.86.  **Feet on blocks**

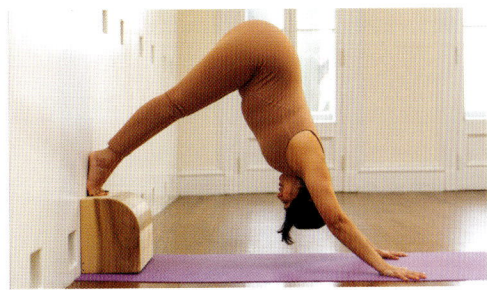

FIGURE 2.87.  **Feet on a Viparīta Karaṇī box**

**Effects** *The heels pressing into the wall moves the root of the thighs farther back, bringing more length to the lumbar spine and lower abdomen.*

### 3. Adho Mukha Śvānāsana with Feet on Blocks or a Stool

Repeat the instructions for Adho Mukha Śvānāsana (pose 1), but place your feet up on blocks (fig. 2.86) or a low stool (fig. 2.87) with the backs of your heels at the wall, legs together. You can experiment with putting the feet on a higher support, which is more challenging but deepens the inverting effect.

**Effects** *As the feet and legs come higher, the pelvic organs are more fully inverted, bringing relief to pelvic organ pressure or prolapse. The legs together bring compactness and stability to the hips and pelvis.*

### 4. Utkaṭāsana with a Block (Fierce Pose)

Stand with your back against a wall and walk your feet about one and a half feet away from the wall—about the length of your thigh—with your feet hips width apart. Place a block at its narrow width between your knees and hug your outer thighs and hips in to squeeze the block. With your palms against the wall, bend your knees and slide your torso down so the knees come to a right angle (figs. 2.88 and 2.89). Keep the entire back body against the wall, including your head. At first, you may not easily be able to come to a right angle, in which case, come down as far as possible while maintaining stability. If your knees come out past your ankles, stand back up and walk your

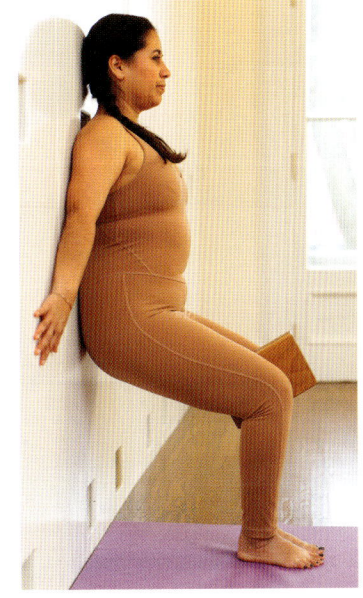

FIGURE 2.88.  **Utkaṭāsana**

feet a little farther from the wall. Lift from your inner arches to the inner knees to the inner thighs, drawing up through the perineum. Bring your tailbone and buttocks down as you draw your navel back toward your spine so the lumbar spine touches the wall. Once this is easily accomplished for a few breaths, try contracting the pelvic floor first (mūla bandha), then draw the navel back and up (uḍḍīyāna bandha), always contracting on the exhalation and releasing on the inhalation. To come up, press your heels into the floor and raise your spine up the wall. At first it may be hard to stay for any length of time. It is better to repeat a few times for short durations as you slowly build up stamina.

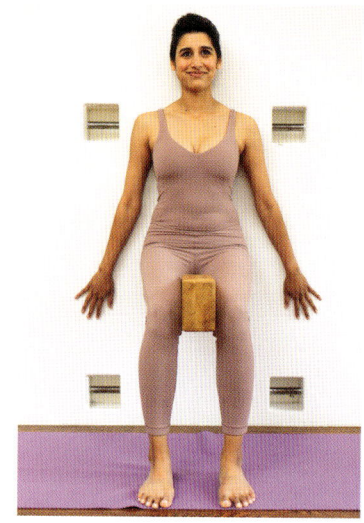

FIGURE 2.89. **Arms down**

## VARIATIONS

GOING DEEPER: Once your legs, hips, and pelvis are stable and engaged, stretch your arms upward with your palms facing forward and press the whole back of your arm into the wall, reaching the sides of your waist upward (fig. 2.90). Take care not to let your lumbar spine push away from the wall when your arms come overhead. This requires more mobility in your shoulders and upper back as well as greater abdominal stability.

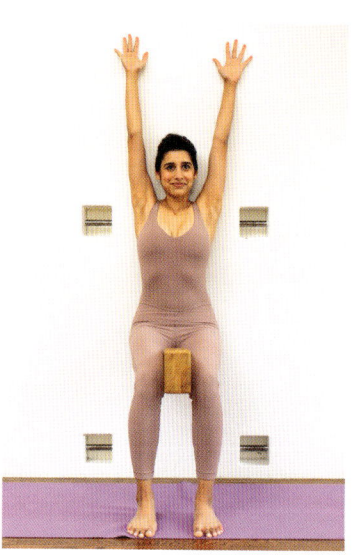

FIGURE 2.90. **Arms up**

***Effects*** *This pose strengthens the legs, inner and outer thighs, and abdomen. It helps to coordinate the pelvic floor and abdominal muscles together, bringing stability to the whole lower torso.*

### 5. Utthita Trikoṇāsana

See fig. 2.91 and Week 4 pose 7 for instructions. Observe deeper mūla bandha and uḍḍīyāna bandha actions, as in Utkaṭāsana. Once stability and lift can be maintained, reach your front hand down to your shin.

## 6. Vīrabhadrāsana II

See fig. 2.92 and Week 4 pose 8 for instructions. Observe deeper mūla bandha and uḍḍīyāna bandha actions, as in Utkaṭāsana.

## 7. Ardha Chandrāsana

See fig. 2.93 and Week 4 pose 9 for instructions. Observe deeper mūla bandha and uḍḍīyāna bandha actions, as in Utkaṭāsana.

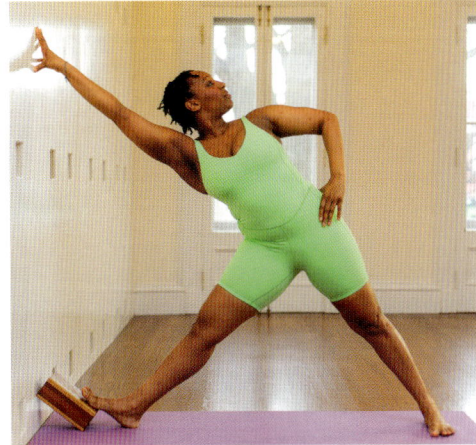

FIGURE 2.91.  **Utthita Trikoṇāsana.**

## 8. Ūrdhva Prasārita Pādāsana 90 Degrees (Upward Extended-Legs Pose)

This pose represents the beginning of doing abdominal work in earnest. A whole treatise could be written on this pose, which, when done with the correct actions, deeply tonifies and massages the abdominal muscles and organs. The abdominal work, started in uḍḍīyāna bandha and in poses like Utkaṭāsana, is continued here, but with the lower back resting on the floor so the abdominal actions will be felt more clearly, and with more support for the spine. It is shown in two stages here so that those with weak abdominals can feel the correct actions before moving on to more strenuous stages of the pose. Overdoing abdominal strengthening, especially for those with weak abdominals, diastasis recti abdominis, or hernias, can actually make symptoms worse,

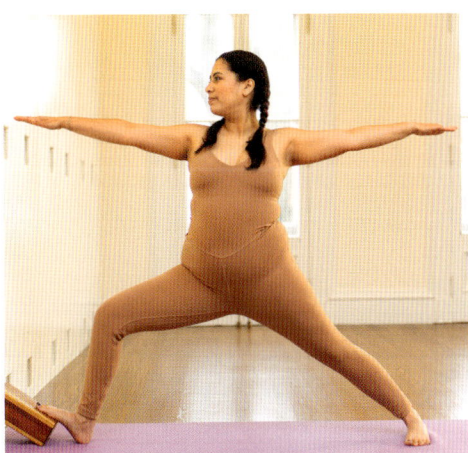

FIGURE 2.92.  **Vīrabhadrāsana II.**

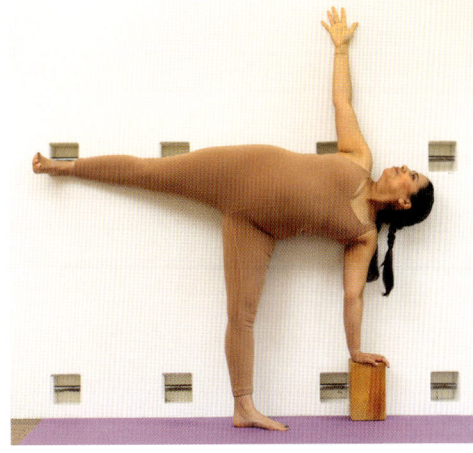

FIGURE 2.93.  **Ardha Chandrāsana.**

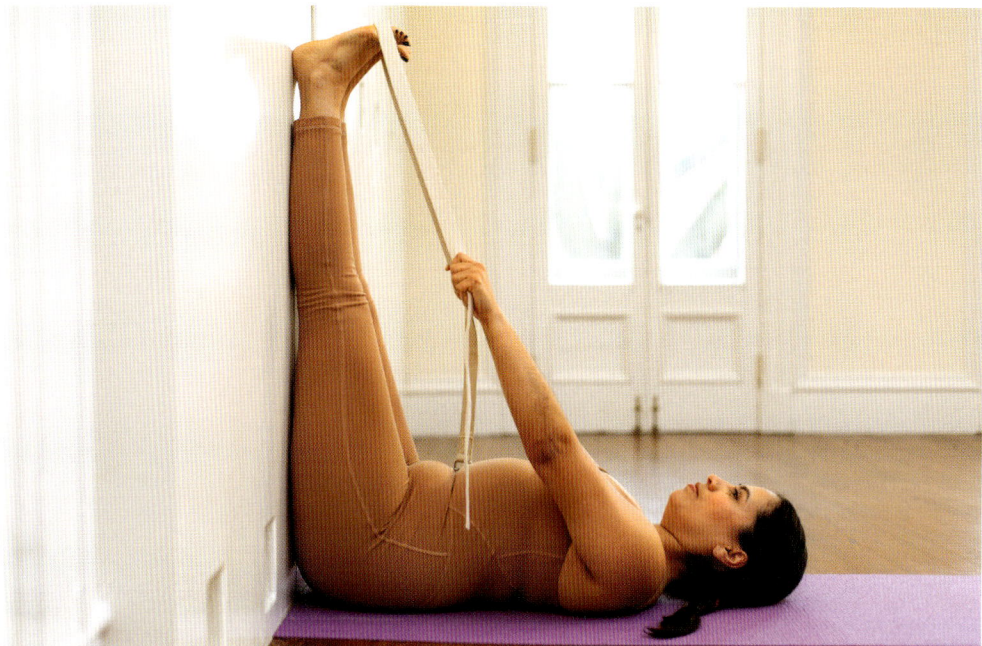

FIGURE 2.94. Ūrdhva Prasārita Pādāsana at the wall with a belt.

so care should be taken to proceed slowly. Be willing to back off, use additional support, and be patient as it can take time for these conditions to heal.

## STAGE 1. AT THE WALL WITH A BELT

Lie down with your legs up the wall and feet together. Place a belt around the ball mounds of your feet and pull back on the belt, keeping your arms straight and your chest lifted, reaching up through the heels (fig. 2.94). Press the entire backs of your legs against the wall, from your buttocks to your heels, and firm the knees and thighs. Draw your outer hips toward the wall and lengthen the sides of your waist away from the wall. Now draw your abdomen toward your spine and up into your chest as in uḍḍīyāna bandha. Hold for a breath or two, and then release and repeat.

## STAGE 2. AT THE WALL, ARMS OVERHEAD

From stage 1, let go of the belt and stretch your arms overhead, maintaining the stretch of your legs and the abdominal action (fig. 2.95). As your arms come overhead, watch that your lumbar spine doesn't overly lift away from the floor. The lumbar spine should remain neutral with a slight curve. If you have weak abdominals or tight shoulders, you may feel that it is challenging to keep the

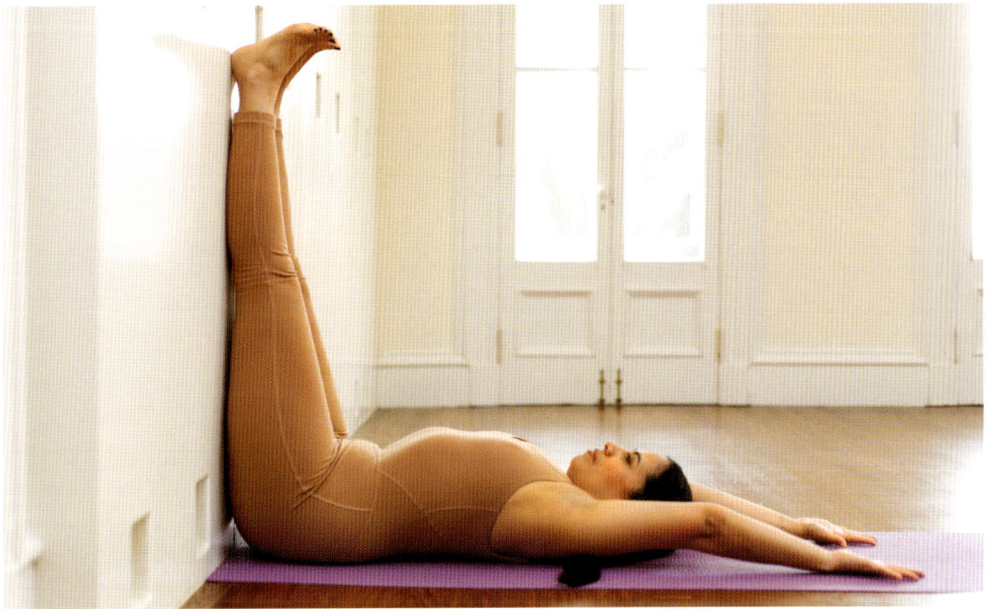

FIGURE 2.95. Ūrdhva Prasārita Pādāsana, at the wall, arms overhead.

abdomen moving back as your arms reach overhead, in which case it's better to attempt to bring the lumbar spine farther down toward the floor, which will help the abdominal muscles contract. If you cannot maintain the abdominal action, it is better to return to stage 1 so as not to put pressure downward on the abdominals and organs or overwork the lumbar spine. Stay for a breath or two, release, and repeat a few times.

*Effects* *This āsana stimulates the transverse abdominis muscles, the deepest layer of abdominal muscles, which work to stabilize the pelvis and lower spine, while simultaneously lengthening all of the abdominal muscles. It massages the organs toward the spine, giving a tonifying effect.*

### 9. SUPTA PĀDĀṄGUṢṬHĀSANA I (SUPINE HAND-TO-BIG-TOE POSE I)

Lie down with your knees bent. Place a belt around the ball of your right foot and stretch your right leg up to 90 degrees, straightening the leg completely. Firm the knee and press the front of your thigh to the back of the thigh as you stretch the calf up to the heel. Without disturbing your right leg, slowly straighten your left leg on the floor (fig. 2.96). Press the whole left leg to the floor, reaching through the inner heel strongly and rolling the inner groin down toward the floor. Draw your outer right thigh away from the side of your waist as you elongate the sides of your waist toward your chest, as in Ūrdhva Prasārita

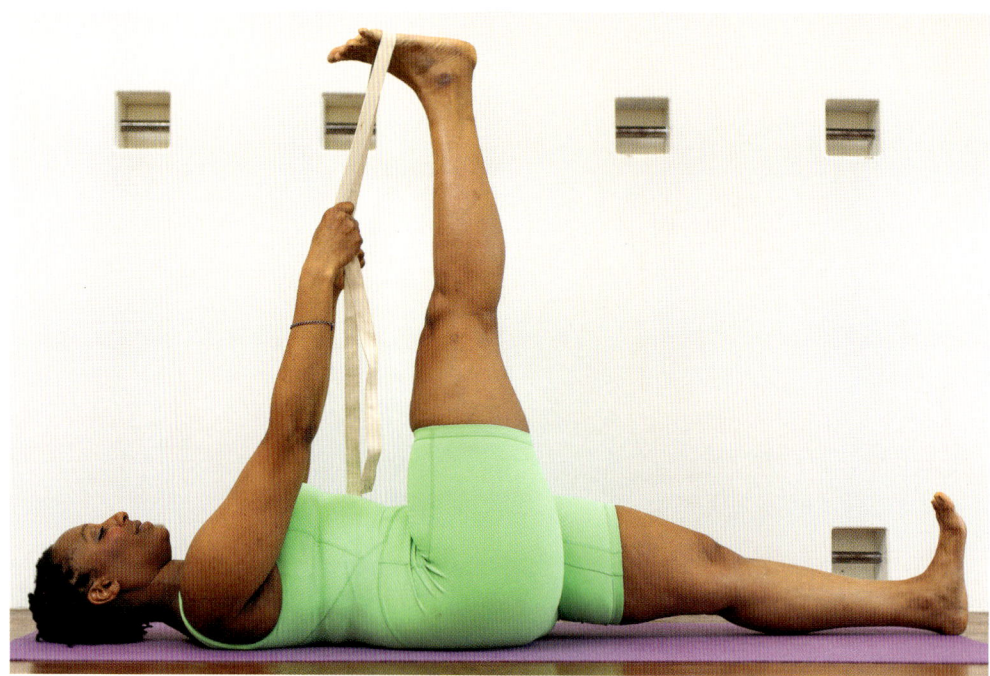

FIGURE 2.96. **Supta Pādāṇguṣṭhāsana I.**

Pādāsana (pose 8). Draw your abdomen back toward your spine and up toward your chest. Hold for twenty to thirty seconds, and then release and repeat on the other side.

## VARIATIONS

TIGHT FRONT GROINS OR ANTERIOR PELVIC TILT: If it is hard to bring the thigh of your bottom leg to the floor while keeping your lumbar spine from overly lifting, place a block under the heel of your bottom leg (fig. 2.97). This helps the pelvis maintain a neutral position rather than tipping forward (anterior tilt).

*Effects Similar to Ūrdhva Prasārita Pādāsana, this pose stimulates the abdominal muscles in a lengthened state. It brings additional mobility to the hamstrings and calves, and creates mobility and compacting in the hip joint.*

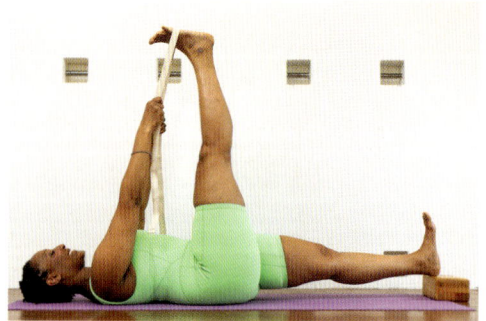

FIGURE 2.97. **Heel on a block**

## 10. SUPTA PĀDĀṄGUṢṬHĀSANA II (SUPINE HAND-TO-BIG-TOE POSE II)

From Supta Pādāṅguṣṭhāsana I, place a folded blanket against your outer thigh as high up against your hip as possible. Keeping your left leg firmly pressing into the floor, slowly stretch your right leg out to the side, keeping the knee firm (fig. 2.98). Maintain the leg at hip level—don't try to pull your foot closer to your shoulder, even if you have the mobility to do so. Only go so far down with your right leg as the groin will safely allow, supporting your outer thigh more if needed with a second blanket or bolster. Keep your right outer hip moving away from the side of your waist. As you stretch from the inner groin to the inner heel, strongly draw your outer thigh and middle buttock (right where the blanket is supporting you) in toward your body, drawing the femur bone strongly into the hip socket. Maintain that, and turn your abdomen toward the left, bringing the left side of your waist and left shoulder down toward the floor. Reach strongly through your left arm to aid the abdominal action. Watch that your left leg and hip stay in their place and don't get pulled toward the right leg. If that happens, back off and come in again, keeping your pelvis evenly weighted on the floor. The emphasis should be on abdominal, pelvic, and hip stability rather than on the stretch of the groin.

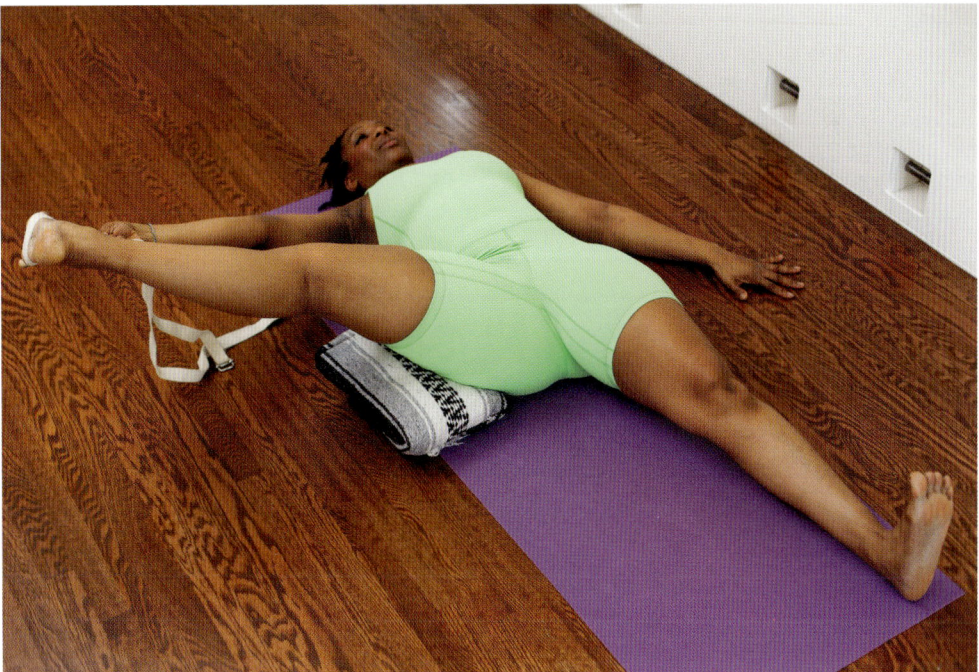

FIGURE 2.98. **Supta Pādāṅguṣṭhāsana II.**

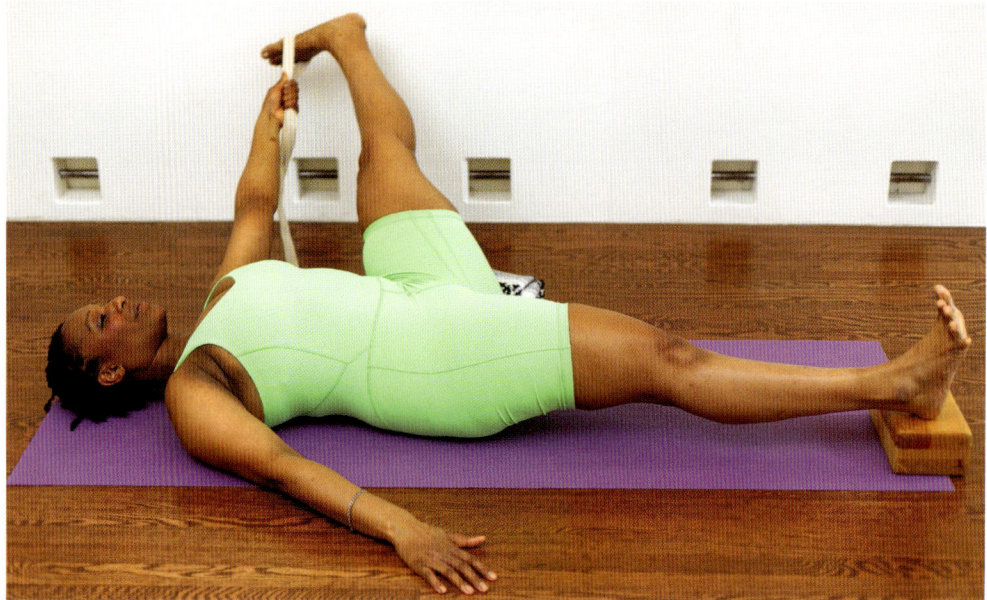

FIGURE 2.99. **Heel on a block**

## VARIATIONS

TIGHT FRONT GROINS OR ANTERIOR PELVIC TILT: If it is hard to bring the thigh of your bottom leg to the floor while keeping your lumbar spine from overly lifting, place a block under the heel of your bottom leg (fig. 2.99). This helps the pelvis maintain a neutral position rather than tipping forward (anterior tilt).

HIP STABILITY: Support the heel of the leg extended out to the side against a wall. As you press your heel into the wall, draw your femur deeper into the socket. If you have a corner available, you can also place your bottom foot against the wall. This will bring a strong compacting action of the joints and a spreading quality of lightness in your abdomen.

***Effects*** *This pose spreads the abdominal and lumbar muscles horizontally as well as vertically, and introduces the turning of the abdominals and organs that will be deepened in later poses.*

## 11. ARDHA ŚĪRṢĀSANA (HALF HEADSTAND)

Śīrṣāsana is a beneficial pose for postpartum healing. Here, Śīrṣāsana is introduced in stages, with the beginner in mind. Individuals who were regularly practicing Śīrṣāsana prior to childbirth need not wait long to resume its practice. In fact, it can be resumed as soon as all bleeding has stopped and once you feel confident in Sarvāṅgāsana. For beginners, however, it can take some time to feel confident practicing this pose, especially when learning on your own. Take time to learn the correct actions of the head, neck, arms, and shoulders, and soon you will be practicing with ease.

Place a sticky mat, folded in quarters, against a wall. Start on your hands and knees. Interlock your fingers to the webbing so that you form a cup shape with your palms. Press the outer edge of your wrists, forearms,

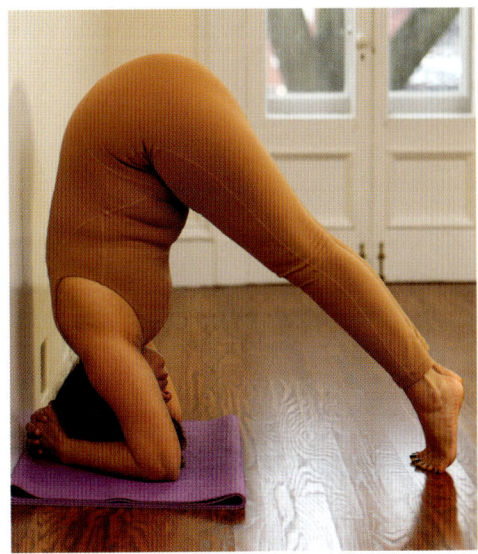

FIGURE 2.100. **Ardha Śīrṣāsana.**

and elbows firmly into the floor. Place the crown of your head down so that the back of your head touches your palms. Close the gap between the back of your head and your palms without letting your wrists roll out. Maintain that, and raise your knees and hips, straightening your legs. Now shift your weight onto your arms and the crown of your head. As you press your forearms down, strongly lift your shoulders up away from your ears and move your upper back in. At first your upper back may want to round toward the wall. Keep your upper back moving away from the wall firmly as you raise your hips higher. Once you are able to maintain this, walk your feet in and lift your shoulders, upper back, and sides of your waist strongly up toward your hips. Stay for one or two breaths, then bend your knees, come down, and rest.

### VARIATIONS

MORE PELVIC LIFT, OR PELVIC ORGAN PROLAPSE: Place a block between your thighs, as in Adho Mukha Śvānāsana.

TIGHT SHOULDERS OR UPPER BACK, OR NECK PAIN: If it is difficult to get your upper back to move in, or there is pain in your neck, you can practice with your head off the floor. Even beginners without neck pain will benefit from the extra mobility in the shoulders that is felt when the head is lifted. Once you are comfortable with this variation, try placing your head down on the floor again without losing the lift of your shoulders and upper back.

**Note:** Those with cervical osteoarthritis, spondylitis, or serious neck injuries may practice this variation as an alternative to Śīrṣāsana, as it helps build upper back and shoulder strength.

## 12. Eka Pāda Ardha Śīrṣāsana (One-Legged Half Headstand)

Once you are steady in Ardha Śīrṣāsana, walk your feet farther in and lift one leg up toward the wall, stretching from your shoulders to your spine to your hips to your raised foot (fig. 2.101). Watch that the hip of your bottom leg doesn't drop downward; rather, lift it strongly and compact your hips. Lower your leg and repeat on the other side, maintaining the lift of your spine. In this stage you will learn to bring mobility to your legs while maintaining steadiness in your head, arms, and shoulders as well as the lift of your spine.

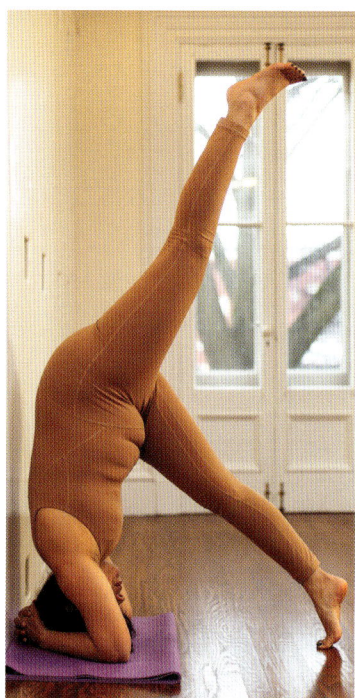

**FIGURE 2.101. Eka Pāda Ardha Śīrṣāsana.**

## 13. Śīrṣāsana (Headstand)

Once you are able to confidently practice the stages discussed so far, it is time to learn to kick up. Keeping your forearms and wrists firmly pressing into the floor, walk your feet in, bend one knee, and swing your opposite leg to the wall, bringing the bottom leg with it (fig. 2.102). You may have to practice kicking a few times to get the rhythm. If your hamstrings are tight, kick up with your knees bent, then straighten your legs.

Now, bring your legs together and strongly stretch up from your shoulders to your buttocks to your heels, stretching your heels higher up the wall, keeping your buttocks lifted and your knees and thighs firm. Roll the fronts of your thighs in and spread the backs of your thighs. Draw your outer hips in and compact the hips as you reach up through your heels. Maintain

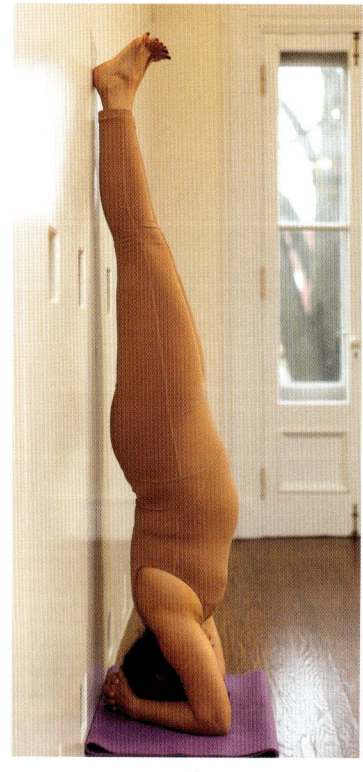

**FIGURE 2.102. Śīrṣāsana.**

the stretch of your whole body and relax your neck, face, and eyes, keeping your brain passive and steady. Stay to your capacity, and then, keeping your shoulders lifted, slowly bring your legs down one at a time, and rest.

At first, postpartum individuals and those with a strong anterior tilt, wide hips, or lower back pain may have difficulty bringing the legs together. The emphasis should be on lifting your buttocks and bringing the tailbone strongly into your body. Once that is achieved, work to gradually bring your legs together, creating compactness in the outer hips, thighs, shins, and ankles.

**Effects** *Śīrṣāsana inverts the organs and helps with prolapse or heaviness in the pelvis, as well as incontinence. It helps to balance the endocrine, respiratory, circulatory, and nervous systems. It quiets and focuses the mind, bringing vitality and renewed energy.*

### 14. Śīrṣāsana with a Block

This is a more intermediate variation for those who can go up with both legs together, or for those who have an assistant who can place the block between the thighs once in the pose. Instructions are given for going up with both knees bent.

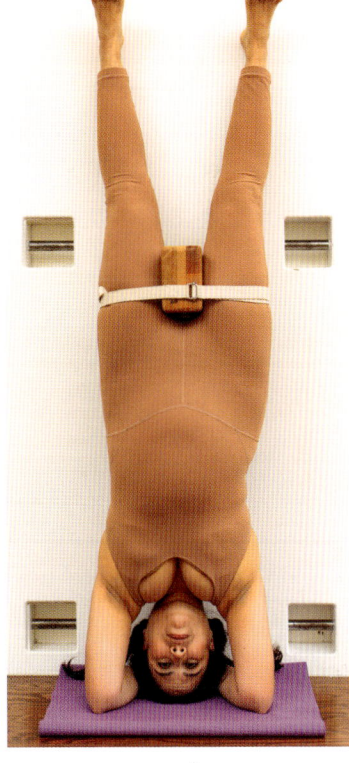

Set up for Śīrṣāsana as in pose 13, placing a block as high up between the thighs as possible, touching the perineum. A belt can be tied around the thighs and the block, or just below the block at the middle of the thighs, for a deeper effect. Walk in and, maintaining the lift of your outer hips and the hugging of the block between your thighs, bring both knees up simultaneously and straighten your legs, feet to the wall (fig. 2.103). Lift your buttocks strongly toward your heels as you stretch your legs up. Turn your inner groins toward the wall to move the block back, but simultaneously move your tailbone in toward the tip of the pubis. Though the actions are the same as those in Tāḍāsana with the block, you may have more sensation and sensitivity to the alignment of your pelvis and the pelvic organs. Feel how your inner thighs are gripping the block. Relax there and try to hug the block from your outer hips,

**FIGURE 2.103.** Śīrṣāsana with a block.

bringing your outer thighs, shins, and ankles closer together. Feel how this creates compactness in the outer body but spreading and softness in the inner body. Stay to your capacity, then bend your knees, come down, and rest.

**Effects** *This variation energizes the legs and creates firmness in the outer hips and buttocks. It brings space to the pelvis and abdomen, creating better alignment of the pelvis and pelvic organs.*

### 15. ŚĪRṢĀSANA WITH KNEES BENT

After you can kick up into Śīrṣāsana with confidence, try practicing this intermediate variation to get better pelvic alignment and abdominal actions.

Set up as in Śīrṣāsana (pose 13). Pull the mat about one and a half feet away from the wall. Come up into Śīrṣāsana and immediately bend your knees, bringing the tips of your toes to the wall with your feet hips width apart. Line up your knees over your hips, legs bent at 90 degrees, thighs vertical (fig. 2.104). If your knees are forward or backward from the line of your hips, come down and adjust the distance to the wall so your knees are directly over your hips. Press your toes into the wall as you lift your tailbone strongly up and slightly draw the top of the pubis toward your navel. Firm the bottom of your buttocks toward the back of your thighs, drawing the hamstrings toward the buttock bones. Notice whether, in bringing the tailbone forward, your thighs also come forward. Work to keep your tailbone in and your buttocks engaged, and press your thighs back again, stretching the fronts of your groins and thighs upward.

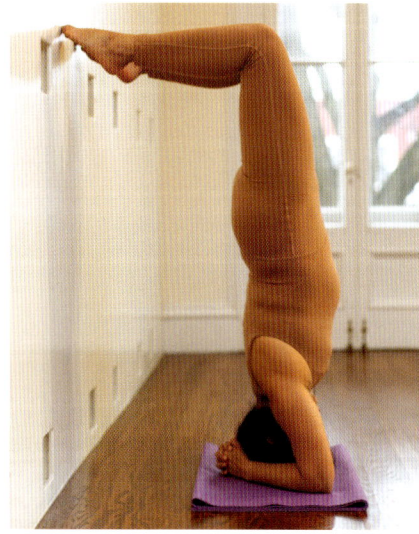 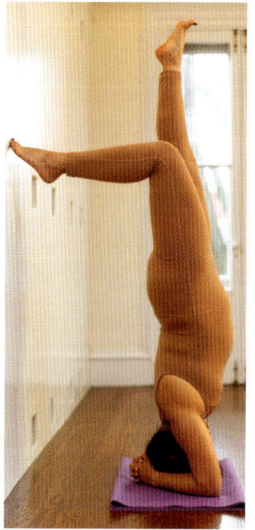 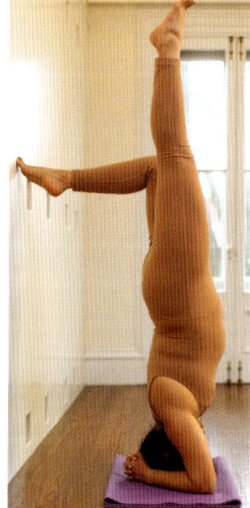

FIGURE 2.104. Śīrṣāsana with knees bent

FIGURE 2.105. Alternating legs

Once you can maintain these actions, try engaging your pelvic floor muscles simultaneously on the exhalation. How does the contraction of your pelvic floor muscles affect the other actions and the feeling in the pose? Once stability is gained, practice stretching one leg up at a time while keeping the other foot pressing into the wall, maintaining the lift of the buttocks. Stay to your capacity, then bring your legs down one at a time and rest.

**Effects** *This variation engages the buttock muscles, hamstrings, and abdomen. The toes on the wall help to create leverage to bring the buttocks up and the tailbone forward, while also stretching the quadriceps and hip flexors. Many postpartum individuals have difficulty with these actions because of the anterior pelvic tilt of pregnancy and the weakness in the abdominals and pelvic floor, and this variation can help to ignite these areas.*

### 16. SĀLAMBA SARVĀṄGĀSANA

See fig. 2.106 and Week 2 pose 6 (stage 3) for instructions.

### 17. ARDHA HĀLĀSANA

See fig. 2.107 and Week 2 pose 7 for instructions.

### 18. ŚAVĀSANA

See fig. 2.108 and Week 1 pose 9 for instructions.

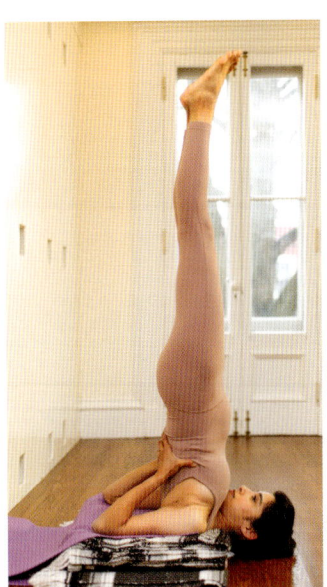

FIGURE 2.106.  **Sālamba Sarvāṅgāsana.**

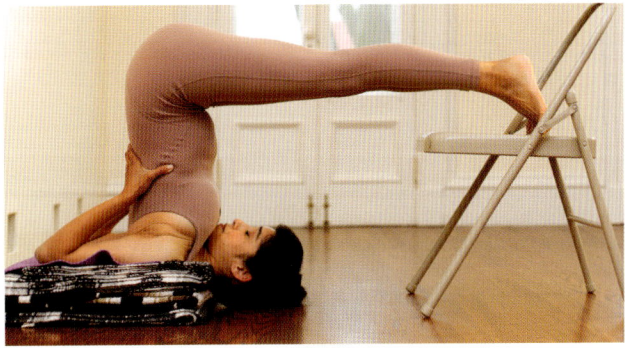

FIGURE 2.107.  **Ardha Hālāsana.**

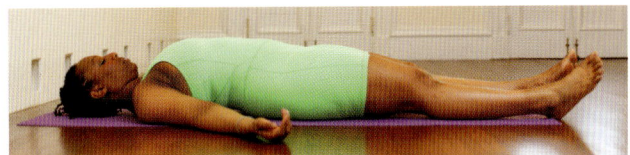

FIGURE 2.108.  **Śavāsana.**

## WEEK 5 FULL SEQUENCE

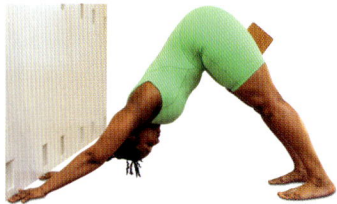

1. Adho Mukha Śvānāsana, hands at the wall (page 123)

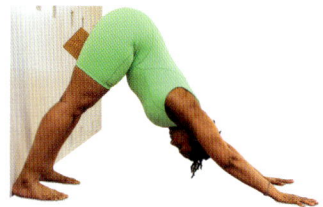

2. Adho Mukha Śvānāsana, heels at the wall (page 124)

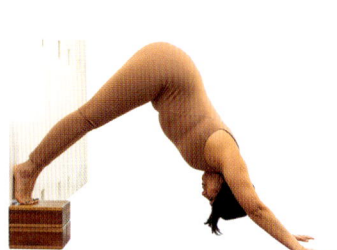

3. Adho Mukha Śvānāsana, feet elevated (page 125)

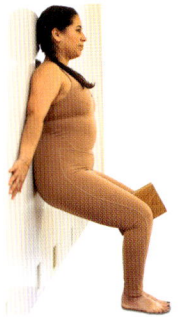

4. Utkaṭāsana (page 125)

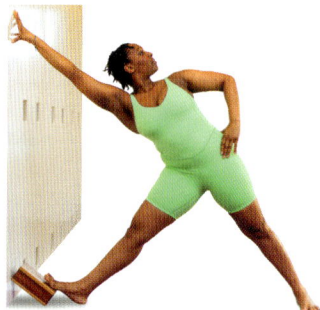

5. Utthita Trikoṇāsana (page 108)

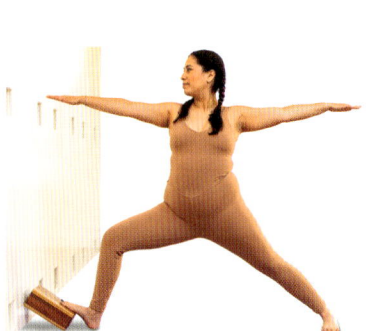

6. Vīrabhadrāsana II (page 110)

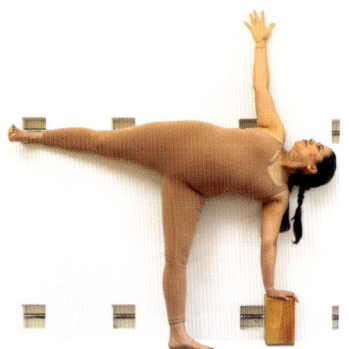

7. Ardha Chandrāsana (page 111)

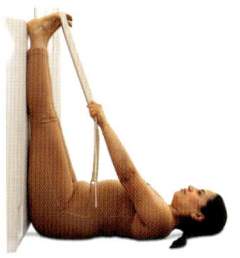

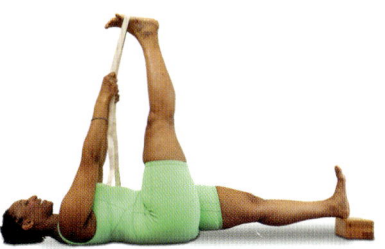

8. Ūrdhva Prasārita Pādāsana (page 127)

9. Supta Pādāṅguṣṭhāsana I (page 129)

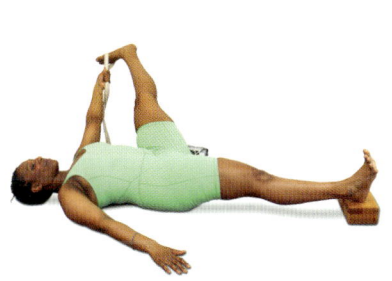

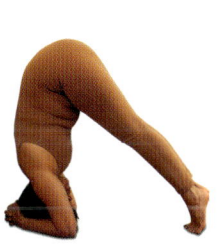

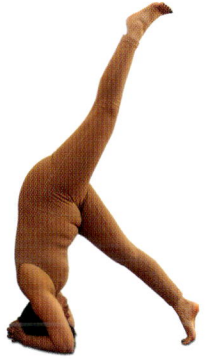

10. Supta Pādāṅguṣṭhāsana II (page 131)

11. Ardha Śīrṣāsana (page 132)

12. Eka Pāda Ardha Śīrṣāsana (page 134)

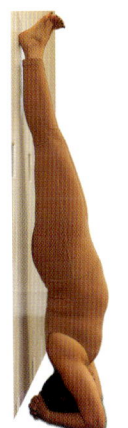

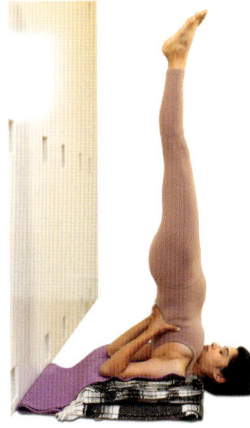

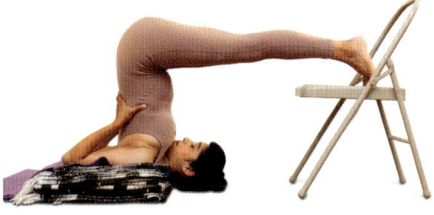

17. Ardha Hālāsana (page 78)

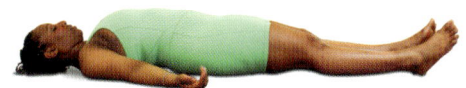

13–15. Śīrṣāsana (page 134)

16. Sālamba Sarvāṅgāsana (page 77)

18. Śavāsana (page 65)

# Week 6
# DEEPENING CONNECTION
## to the CORE

In the previous sequence we began incorporating an abdominal lifting action, sometimes referred to as uḍḍīyāna bandha, into a variety of different poses. Now that we have an awareness of this primary movement, we can begin our deeper abdominal work. The work here in this sequence focuses on learning how to engage the transverse abdominis (TA) muscles, which are the deepest layer of abdominal muscles (see "The Abdominal Container" in chapter 1). The TA muscles run in a horizontal direction, creating a stabilizing band that aids in pelvic and lower spinal stability. You should become familiar with how to feel these muscles engaging, and learn to identify whether there are imbalances. Once these muscles are strong, other abdominal work can be deepened.

Additionally, you may feel in this sequence the strengthening and lengthening effect of the poses on the iliopsoas muscles (see "The Abdominal Container" and "The Respiratory Diaphragm" in chapter 1). These muscles are an important part of the posterior abdominal wall and can become shortened during pregnancy. Composed of three muscles, the psoas major and minor and the iliacus, they run from the 12th thoracic vertebra and lumbar vertebrae (psoas) and the inner surface of the ilium (iliacus) and then join and run through the back of the pelvis, over the hip joint, and insert on the inner femur. They are the only muscles that connect your legs directly to your spine! Additionally, the psoas muscle fibers cross with the attachments of the respiratory diaphragm, making breathing an important part of any abdominal action.

Don't expect to perform this entire sequence your first time practicing. The poses here are given in stages and need not be done all at once, especially for those who are beginners, have young children, or have limited time. In addition, the poses here are sequential and become more challenging. If the actions are not felt or are lost as you progress, return to earlier poses on the sequence and stay with those for a few weeks before attempting the harder poses again. Though progress may seem slow at first, approaching this sequence with patience and compassion will yield better results and create less possibility of injury.

## ISOLATING THE TRANSVERSE ABDOMINIS MUSCLES

As discussed in chapter 1, the transverse abdominis (TA) muscles are the deepest of the four layers of abdominal muscle, and it is important to learn to engage and isolate these muscles because they influence intra-abdominal pressures, allow for efficient load transfer from one part of the body to another, and are a building block for developing core stability.

1. Lie on your back with knees bent and feet flat on the ground.

2. Place your fingertips on the front points of your pelvic bones on each side, and slide them down and in to rest on the soft tissue inside the bones. Beneath your fingertips are your TA muscles.

3. Visualize the horizontally oriented muscle fibers on each side of your body.

4. Maintain light pressure through your finger pads and exhale steadily with sound, saying "shh" as if you're quieting a baby.

5. As you make this sound, your TA muscles contract and you will feel a subtle tension generated beneath your finger pads. You may also try drawing your front hip points in toward each other, narrowing the space between them.

6. When your exhale is complete, inhale and feel the TA muscles relax beneath your fingertips.

During your exhale, check that your abdomen does not push out or suck in strongly as this might mean that other abdominal muscles are also engaging.

When learning to strengthen the abdominal muscles, you should proceed slowly and with caution so that adverse effects are avoided. Putting too much pressure on abdominal and pelvic organs or on the muscles themselves can be counterproductive. This is especially true for those recovering from cesarean section or other abdominal surgery, those with a separation of the rectus abdominis muscle (diastasis recti abdominis), pelvic organ prolapse, or hernias (see chapter 3). Abdominal āsanas can provide great assistance to those with lower back pain; however, you must practice intelligently to ensure that the correct muscles are engaging and initiating the actions so that further overwork in the spinal and lumbar muscles is avoided.

Those who are postpartum should wait ten to twelve weeks before beginning abdominal work, and even then should proceed very slowly, only doing a few repetitions at first. Those who have had a cesarean delivery should wait twelve to sixteen weeks postpartum. The poses in this sequence are contraindicated for menstruation, with the exception of Setubandha Sarvāṅgāsana.

## Sequence of Āsanas: Week 6

### 1. Ardha Setubandha (Half Bridge Pose)

Traditionally, Setubandha is taught as a strong chest opening pose, but here the focus is solely on the pelvic movement (hence the term *ardha,* which means "half"). The upper back and shoulder blades are fully on the floor as opposed to lifted. This brings more pelvic and abdominal awareness, and may spotlight areas of weakness to the more seasoned practitioner, especially in backward extension poses. This pose is taught here in many stages, with a focus on engaging the deepest layer of abdominal muscle, the TA muscles. Before proceeding, it is best to first try isolating these muscles so that you can feel whether they are engaging as you progress through the stages of Ardha Setubandha.

### STAGE 1. FEET ON THE FLOOR

Once you can feel your TA muscles, it is time to add in some further actions. Lie on the floor with your knees bent, heels about six inches from your buttocks, and your feet hips width apart (fig. 2.109). Press your palms down by your sides, and on an exhalation, engage your buttocks, move your tailbone into your body,

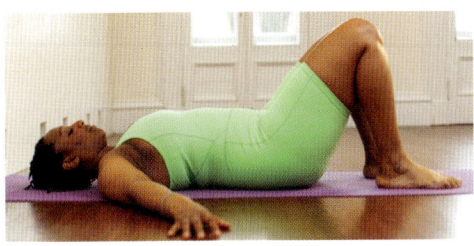

FIGURE 2.109.  Neutral pelvis

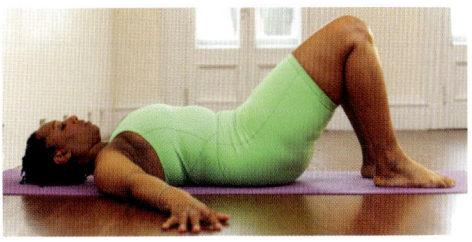

FIGURE 2.110.  With posterior tilt and abdominal engagement

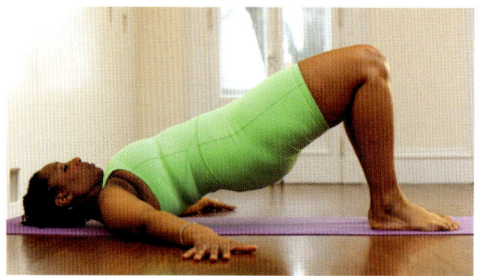

FIGURE 2.111.  **Lifting the pelvis**

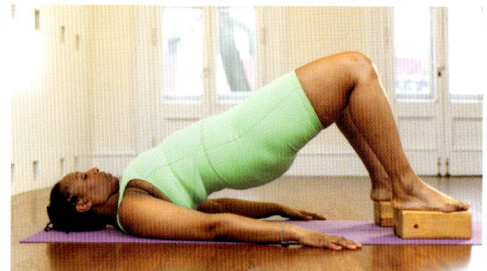

FIGURE 2.112.  **Lifting the pelvis with feet on blocks**

and tilt your pelvis in a posterior direction while keeping your pelvis on the floor (fig. 2.110). Inhale and release. Repeat this a few times until you feel your buttocks, hamstrings, and deeper abdominal muscles engaging.

At first your TA muscles may be hard to feel, or you may feel one side more than the other. You may also feel that other muscles quickly take over. With time, you will develop better awareness. The emphasis should be on developing this awareness and evenly engaging within a small range of motion, rather than trying to get a higher bridge shape. Once this can be felt, attempt contracting the pelvic floor muscles, holding for a few breaths, and then releasing and relaxing.

Once you can feel your TA muscles engaging, proceed to raise your buttocks off of the floor a small distance (fig. 2.111). Strongly lift your tailbone up and in, bringing your buttocks toward the backs of your thighs. Especially feel the bottom of the buttock nearest the upper thigh and lift from there. Keep the lumbar spine long. Notice whether you have a tendency to try to lift from the lumbar spine. In the beginning, don't try to lift to your maximum distance—only lift as far as you can, maintaining the lift from the bottom buttock. Stay for one or two breaths, then release and come down. Rest, and then repeat several times.

### VARIATIONS

BACK PAIN: Place your feet on two flat blocks (fig. 2.112). This brings more length to the lumbar spine and better lifts the pelvis.

***Effects*** *As the tailbone lifts, your navel will move closer to the spine and the TA muscles will engage. This stage brings stability to the "core" and the whole pelvic region. It strengthens the buttocks and hamstrings, which brings stability to the hip joints.*

## STAGE 2. ALTERNATING HEELS

From stage 1, lift one heel off of the floor, keeping the other heel firm, and maintain the buttock, tailbone, and abdominal actions (fig. 2.113). See that your pelvis stays level and doesn't "tip" as the heel is raised. It can be helpful to keep your fingertips on your hip bones and feel whether the pelvis is level. You should observe how the TA muscles of the opposite side engage as your heel is raised. Hold for just one or two seconds, then lower that heel, and repeat on the other side (fig. 2.114). Alternate several times, then release and rest. Take note of any differences or imbalances. It might be helpful to consider the following:

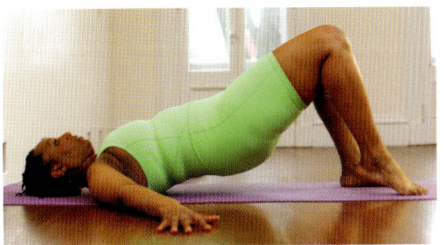

FIGURE 2.113. **Alternating heels.**

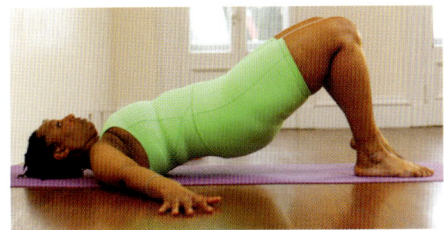

FIGURE 2.114. **Alternating heels.**

Am I able to keep my hips level?

Does one side drop more than the other?

Do I feel weakness in any other muscles?

If you are not able to maintain the evenness of your pelvis, an easier way to practice is to simply alternate pressing your feet down, so that both feet remain completely on the floor. The foot that is pressing down will take more of the weight of the pose, and the TA muscles on that side will engage more.

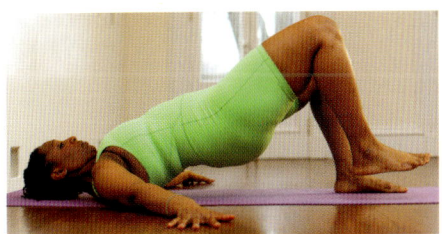

FIGURE 2.115. **Alternating feet.**

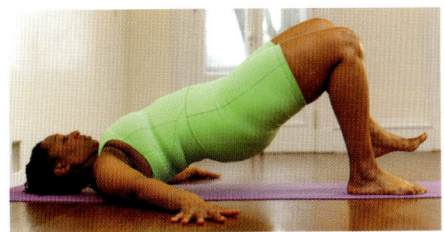

FIGURE 2.116. **Alternating feet.**

## STAGE 3. ALTERNATING LIFTING FEET

For a deeper challenge, now try lifting one foot completely off the floor a few inches. Again, the pelvis should stay absolutely stable while engaging the buttocks, hamstrings, and abdominal muscles on the side with the foot that's pressing into the floor (figures 2.115 and 2.116). The focus should be on the stabilizing side and not on raising the opposite foot higher. Stay for one breath, then lower the foot and repeat on the other side. Practice several repetitions per your capacity, then lower the buttocks and rest.

### 2. Ūrdhva Prasārita Pādāsana 90 Degrees

Like Ardha Setubandha, this pose is given in stages to create stability and sensitivity in the practitioner. While the classic pose is deeply strengthening, it can be too much for the beginner or those who are recovering from childbirth. Again, keep the emphasis on minimal action and range of motion with maximum awareness.

Set up as in Ūrdhva Prasārita Pādāsana in Week 5, with the buttocks a few inches away from the wall and the heels at the wall (fig. 2.117). Repeat all the same actions, and keeping your knees firm, raise one heel off the wall, bringing your leg to 90 degrees (figures 2.118 and 2.119). Watch that your leg doesn't swing and come past 90 degrees. Observe your abdomen and lumbar spine. Your navel should continue to move toward your spine, and your lumbar spine should stay close to the floor. Now slowly lower your foot back down, and repeat on the other side. Observe:

Are there any imbalances or differences?

Does one side feel easier than the other?

Does this connect with any imbalance in the pelvic floor muscles?

Now, keeping both legs and feet together, bring your legs off the wall together (fig. 2.120). You may notice that this is significantly harder than bringing up one leg at a time. Watch that your abdomen doesn't "puff" forward and that your lumbar spine doesn't overly arch. Maintaining your navel toward the spine and up toward the chest (uḍḍīyāna bandha), slowly lower your legs back to the wall. Repeat several times, then bend your knees and rest.

### VARIATIONS

If you feel ready to move your legs away from the wall but are losing the length of the abdomen, you can hold on to something sturdy overhead, like the low bars on a rope wall (fig. 2.121), or the underside of a couch or other heavy piece of furniture.

**Effects** *This pose engages the transverse abdominis muscles and abdominals while also lengthening them. The iliopsoas muscles (hip flexors) are strengthened. It massages the organs toward the spine, giving a tonifying effect.*

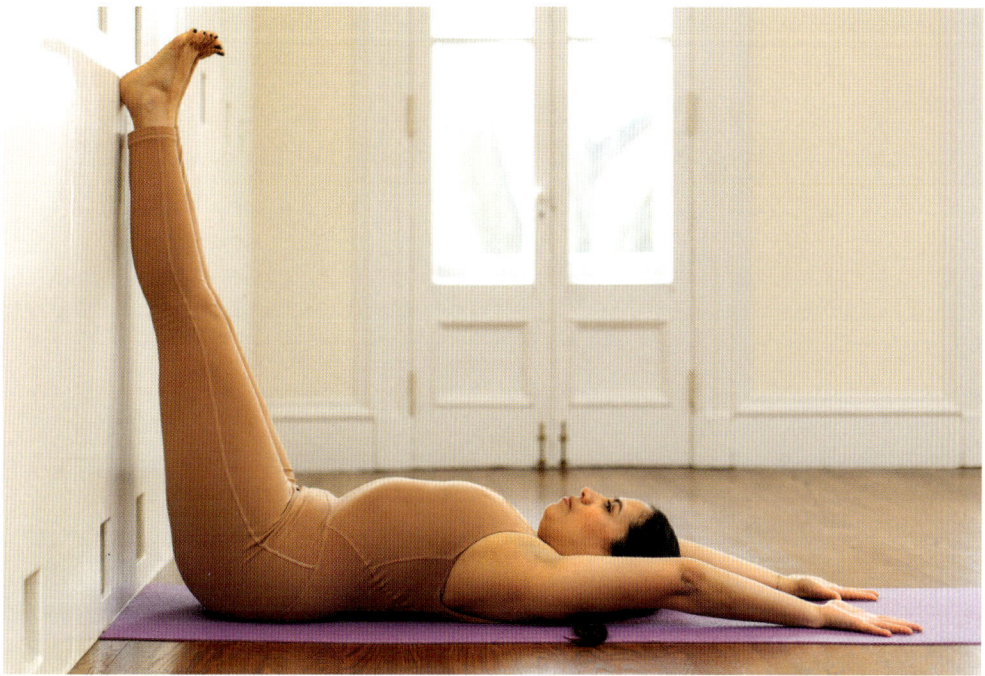

FIGURE 2.117.  Ūrdhva Prasārita Pādāsana, 90 degrees, feet at the wall.

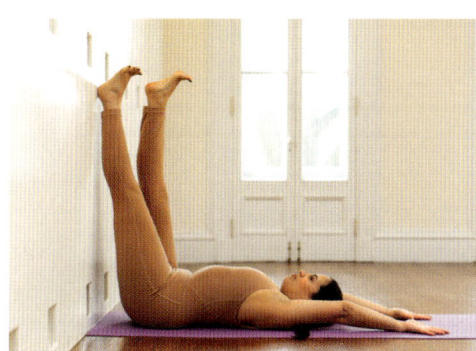

FIGURE 2.118.  Alternating feet off the wall

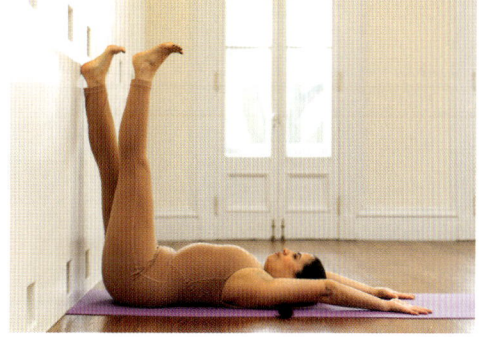

FIGURE 2.119.  Alternating feet off the wall

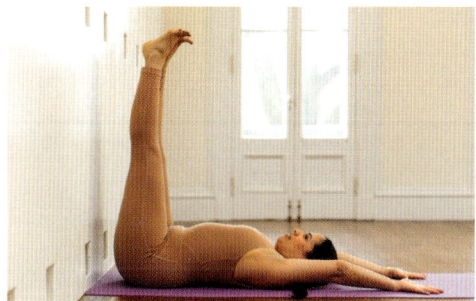

FIGURE 2.120.  Both feet off the wall

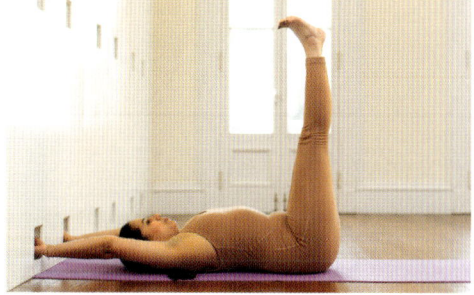

FIGURE 2.121.  Arms anchored overhead

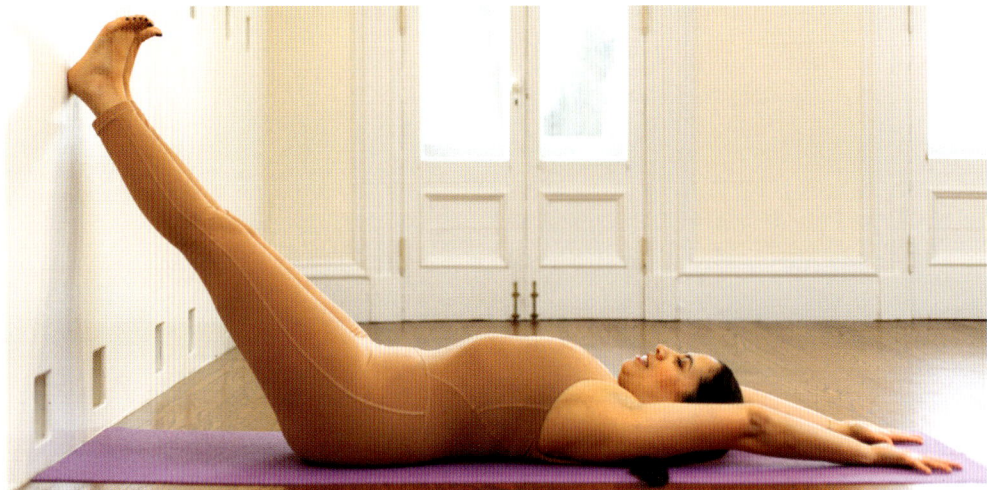

FIGURE 2.122. Ūrdhva Prasārita Pādāsana, 60 degrees, feet at the wall.

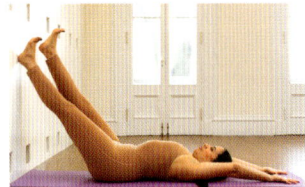

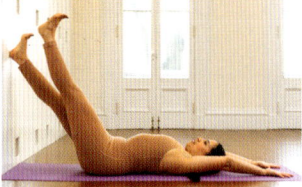

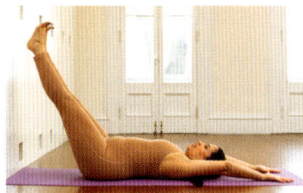

FIGURE 2.123. Alternating feet off the wall

FIGURE 2.124. Alternating feet off the wall

FIGURE 2.125. Both feet off the wall

### 3. Ūrdhva Prasārita Pādāsana 60 Degrees

Once your are stable in the previous stage, bring your buttocks farther away from the wall and repeat the instructions, bringing the feet to 60 degrees (figures 2.122 to 2.125). This builds up more strength in the abdominals and iliopsoas muscles.

### 4. Ūrdhva Prasārita Pādāsana 30 Degrees

Bring the buttocks farther away from the wall and repeat the instructions, bringing the feet to 30 degrees (figures 2.126 to 2.129). As this is the most challenging variation, this pose requires tremendous strength in the abdominals and hip flexors.

## VARIATIONS

Each stage works slightly different areas of the abdominal muscles and hip flexors, as they involve both raising and lowering the legs. If the more challenging stages aren't accessible, you may still bring your buttocks away from the wall and practice raising your foot off the wall only one or two inches, and then releasing and repeating on the other side. Eventually you can build up to bringing both feet off the wall

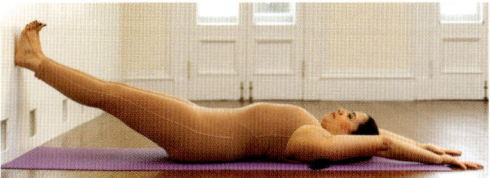

FIGURE 2.126. Ūrdhva Prasārita Pādāsana, 30 degrees, feet at the wall.

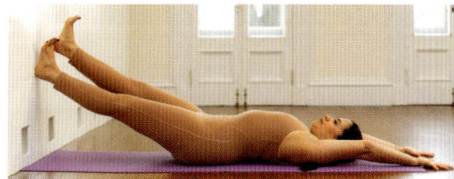

FIGURE 2.127. Alternating feet off the wall

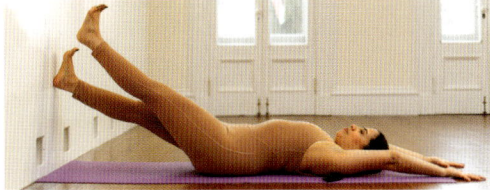

FIGURE 2.128. Alternating feet off the wall

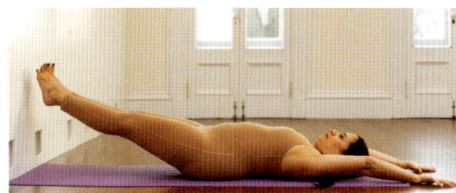

FIGURE 2.129. Both feet off the wall

momentarily. At first, you may only be able to sustain it for one or two seconds. It is better to repeat a few times rather than trying to hold for a long period.

## 5. Paripūrṇa Nāvāsana with Knees Bent, Hands on the Floor (Full Boat Pose)

As in the previous poses, Nāvāsana is given here in stages in order to make the correct actions accessible to those who are postpartum, recovering from abdominal surgery, or experiencing other issues in which the abdominals may be weakened and compromised.

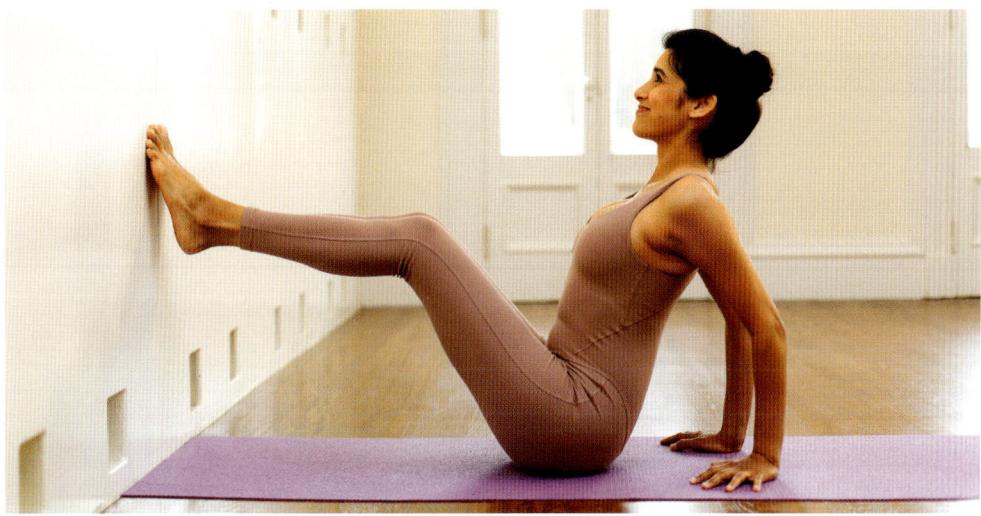

FIGURE 2.130. Paripūrṇa Nāvāsana with knees bent.

### STAGE 1. KNEES BENT, FEET AT THE WALL

Sit with your knees bent, about two feet from the wall, feet facing the wall. Place your palms by the sides of your hips, fingers pointing toward your feet. Now pressing your palms down, point your elbows back and lean back slightly. As you lean back, watch that your lumbar spine doesn't drop toward the floor. Lift your lumbar spine and back ribs up to keep your weight on the buttock bones. There should be no pressure on the sacrum. Now draw your abdomen back and up toward your chest as in uḍḍīyāna bandha. Move your shoulder blades down your back and press them into the back ribs in order to lift your chest. Stay for a breath or two, maintaining these actions. Some may find even this initial stage challenging; if this is the case, stay here and work on this preparatory stage for several weeks until strength is built. Once this is achieved, walk your feet up the wall one at a time, knees bent, feet in line with your knees and legs together. Observe what happens in your pelvis, abdomen, and lumbar spine. Work to maintain stability in these areas as your legs come up. Stay for two or three breaths, gradually working up to a minute. Then release and stretch your legs out.

### STAGE 2. KNEES BENT, ALTERNATING FEET

From stage 1, raise one foot off the wall, keeping your pelvis, abdomen, and lumbar spine stable (fig. 2.131). Hold for just one or two seconds, and then return your foot to the wall. Repeat on the opposite side. Alternate several times, then release and stretch your legs out.

### STAGE 3. KNEES BENT, BOTH FEET OFF THE WALL

Once stability is maintained in stage 2, bring both feet off the wall, legs pressing firmly together (fig. 2.132). Observe that your weight doesn't shift back to the sacrum; rather, lift the top of your sacrum, lumbar spine, and back ribs up.

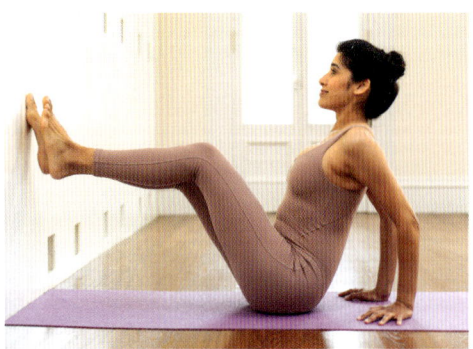

FIGURE 2.131. **Alternating feet.**

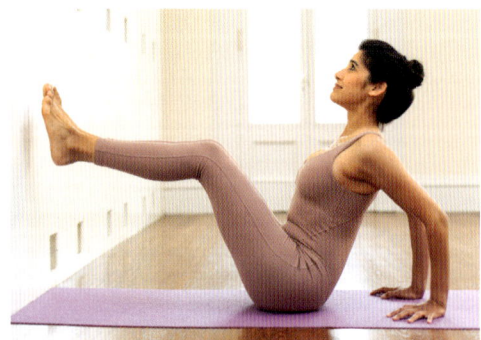

FIGURE 2.132. **Both feet off wall.**

From here, you may also practice bringing less and less weight to your hands, holding the pose from your abdominals, lumbar spine, and hips. From here you may begin to practice contracting the pelvic floor muscles to see if that brings you more stability in the pose. The pelvic floor contraction may give you more of the feeling of lifting and "floating" in your boat.

**Effects** *This abdominal āsana tones the abdomen and lumbar muscles. It teaches the synchronized lift of the posterior (back) and anterior (front) sides of the body.*

### 6. Paripūrṇa Nāvāsana with Legs Straight, Hands on the Floor

### STAGE 1. FEET AT THE WALL

Once the previous stages are achieved, stretch your legs straight up the wall with your heels pressing the wall and your legs together. Your feet should be approximately in line with your shoulders or a little bit higher (fig. 2.133). Roll your thighs inward, firm your knees, and reach from your inner legs through your inner heels. Engage your buttocks toward the backs of your thighs without rocking your weight back onto the sacrum. Rather, lift straight up off the tip of the tailbone. Maintaining the abdominal and lumbar lift, bring your shoulder blades down your back as you lift your chest. Keep your throat, neck, and face quiet. Stay for two or three breaths, then release, and rest. This can be repeated several times.

### STAGE 2. ALTERNATING LEGS

From stage 1, raise one heel slightly off the wall. Maintaining the stability of your pelvis, firm the knee of your raised leg as you reach strongly through your inner heel (fig. 2.134). Release and repeat on the other side. At first, it will be hard to keep the knee of your raised leg straight. However, over time your leg

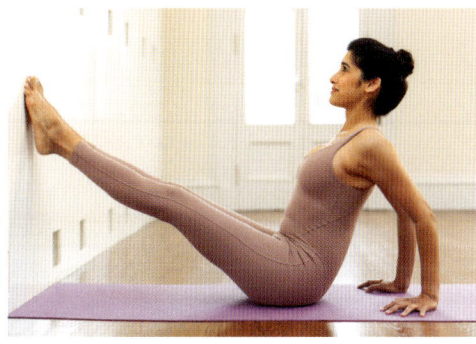

FIGURE 2.133. Paripūrṇa Nāvāsana, with legs straight.

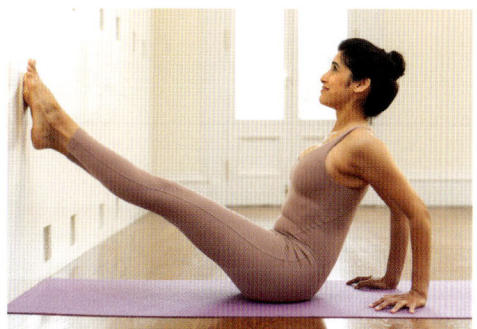

FIGURE 2.134. Paripūrṇa Nāvāsana, alternating feet.

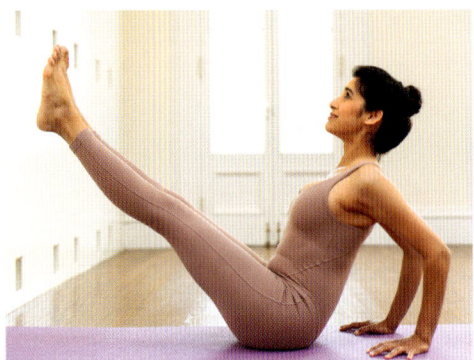

FIGURE 2.135. Paripūrṇa Nāvāsana, both feet off wall.

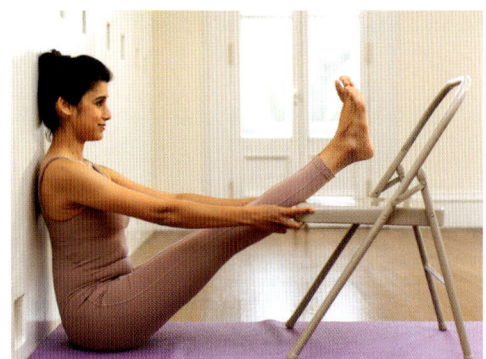

FIGURE 2.136. Paripūrṇa Nāvāsana with a chair.

muscles will strengthen. If your hamstrings are tight, move a few inches farther away from the wall.

## STAGE 3. BOTH FEET OFF THE WALL

From stage 1, firm your legs together and simultaneously raise both heels off the wall (fig. 2.135). If that is too difficult, or if your pelvis rocks back, try bringing your feet off the wall with your knees bent (as in stage 3 of the previous pose), and then straighten them. Reach through your inner legs to the inner heels as you firm your outer thighs in toward each other. Keep your buttocks engaged and moving into your body. Lift up from your pelvic floor to create lightness in the spine. Begin to lessen the weight on your hands. Feel the whole structure of your pelvis, like the bottom of the boat holding the organs and floating above the water. Stay for up to one minute, then release and rest.

*Effects* *This pose strengthens the abdomen and spine. It also strengthens the iliopsoas and quadriceps, especially the area around the inner knee. It brings compactness to the hips and buttocks.*

### 7. Paripūrṇa Nāvāsana Variation with a Chair

Sit with your back toward the wall, buttocks slightly away from the wall, and lean back so that your back ribs are held by the wall. Bend your knees and bring your calves up onto a chair seat. Reach forward and hold the sides of the chair (fig. 2.136), pulling it toward you as you draw your upper arms into the sockets and lift your chest. Lift from the lower spine and abdomen to lift your chest up. With your legs together, stretch the legs up, reaching through the inner legs to your inner heels, calves resting on the chair. If you are not able to straighten your legs, or your spine is rounding, move the chair a few inches away from the wall. For those with tight hamstrings, the chair may also need to be farther from the wall. If in moving the chair farther away you can no longer reach it with your hands, loop a belt around the back of the chair and hold the belt in your hands. Stay for up to one minute, then release and rest.

**Effects** *This variation gives more of a massaging action to the abdominal and pelvis organs as the legs come closer to the spine. One begins to learn the reaching and drawing-in actions of the arms and shoulders. The upper back and head rest on the wall, bringing quietness to the throat and the brain. This variation may be helpful to those who've had a cesarean section or those recovering from abdominal surgery as it teaches the correct actions without overworking.*

### 8. Paripūrṇa Nāvāsana Variation Holding a Belt

Sit with knees bent and loop a belt around the balls of your feet. Lean back slightly, draw your abdomen back and up, compact your hips, firm your legs together, and raise your feet off the floor with your knees bent. Balance here for a moment, keeping the back and front body lifted and your arms moving into the sockets as you pull on the strap with two straight arms. Now stretch through your inner legs to the inner heels and inner ball mounds of your feet and raise your legs, straightening your legs completely. Firm your knees and thighs and use the tension of the belt to lift your chest more. Stay centered on your buttock bones and balance. Hold for two or three breaths, then bend your legs and come down.

**Effects** *This pose creates firmness in the knees, thighs, buttocks, abdomen, and spine. The belt helps teach the arms to draw in toward the sockets, helping to lift the chest. The coordination of the arms and legs is improved, and you begin to feel your center of gravity as the balance is achieved.*

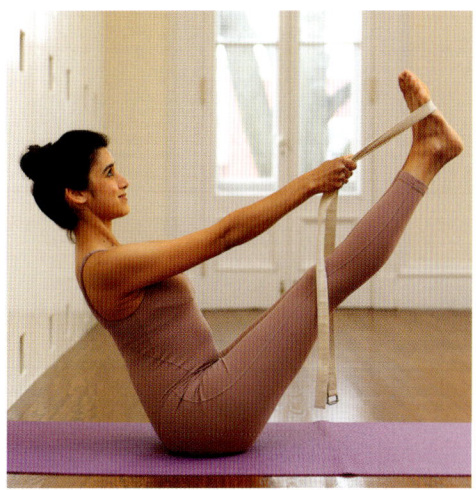

**FIGURE 2.137.** **Paripūrṇa Nāvāsana with a belt.**

## 9. Nirālamba Supta Pādāṅguṣṭhāsana I (Unsupported Supine Hand-to-Big-Toe Pose I)

Traditionally, Supta Pādāṅguṣṭhāsana is taught holding the big toe or foot with the hand or a belt. *Nirālamba* means unsupported, and in this variation, no support is used in order to teach the leg to hold itself and to maintain its connection with the hip joint and pelvis. This version of Supta Pādāṅguṣṭhāsana should only be attempted once the previous abdominal poses in both Weeks 5 and 6 are achieved as it requires deeper strength and stability in the pelvis and abdomen.

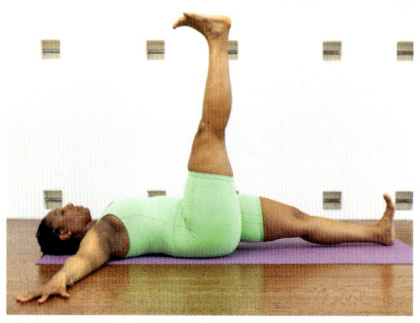

FIGURE 2.138. **Nirālamba Supta Pādāṅguṣṭhāsana I.**

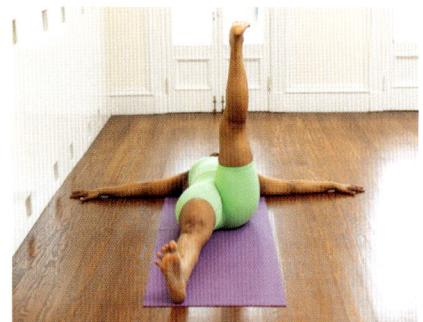

FIGURE 2.139. **Alternate view.**

Lie down with knees bent, and extend your arms out to your sides in line with your shoulders, palms facing down. Stretch your right leg vertically up toward the ceiling, as in Supta Pādāṅguṣṭhāsana I (pose 9 in Week 5). Extend your left leg out on the floor, pressing the whole back of your thigh to the floor. Descend your left inner groin down as you reach from your inner leg through your inner heel and inner ball mound of your foot. Your raised leg may be hard to straighten at first. Firm the front of your thigh to the bone, especially the area just above the knee, and reach strongly through your heel and the inner ball mound of your foot. Keeping your legs well extended, reach your arms overhead with your palms facing up, and press the backs of your hands, your arms, and your shoulders into the floor. Lengthen your lumbar spine while simultaneously bringing your abdomen back toward your spine and up into your chest. Move the root of your right thigh away from your waist and elongate both sides of your waist toward your hands. Stay for two or three breaths, then release and repeat on the other side.

### VARIATIONS

If you have WIDE HIPS OR LOWER BACK PAIN, you may need to move your bottom leg farther out to the side so that your outer heel is more in line with your outer hip.

HIP PAIN IN THE BOTTOM LEG: Move your bottom heel wider and support it on a low block.

***Effects*** *This pose tones the abdomen, outer hips, thighs, and knees. It brings firmness to the pelvis and teaches how to stretch and move the legs while maintaining pelvic and abdominal stability.*

### 10. Nirālamba Supta Pādāṅguṣṭhāsana II (Unsupported Supine Hand-to-Big-Toe Pose II)

Start in the previous pose. Now stretch your arms out to your sides in line with your shoulders, palms facing down, and slowly reach your raised leg out to the side, keeping your heel in line with your hip. Start very slowly as you will not be able to go as far as you were able to with the support of the blanket and belt in Week 5, pose 10. As your leg travels to the side, watch that your pelvis doesn't get pulled to that side. Reach from your inner groin to the inner heel of your raised leg, but draw back from your outer thigh to your hip and strongly suck the outer femur into the socket. Your medial buttock should strongly engage and support the leg bone; think about what the blanket was doing for you in this pose in Week 5. Move your outer hip away from the side of your waist and elongate your waist toward your chest. Keep your bottom leg reaching away from you and press the root of your thigh down to keep the left side of your pelvis on the floor. Observe evenness in the weight on both sides of the sacrum and pelvis.

Now turn your pubic bone and lower abdomen away from your raised leg and bring the opposite side of your waist closer toward the floor. Both shoulders should stay evenly pressing on the floor. Check to see that there is a straight line from the inner heel of your bottom leg to the center of your pubis, navel, sternum, and head. Stay for two or three breaths, then bring your inclined leg up, bend your knees, and

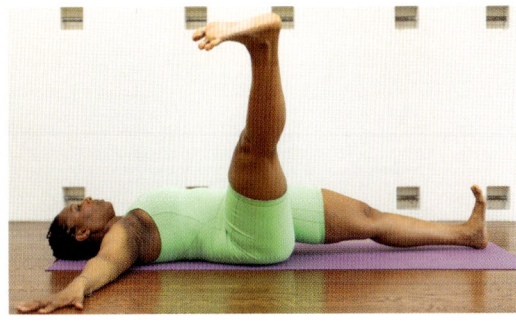

**FIGURE 2.140.** Nirālamba Supta Pādāṅguṣṭhāsana II.

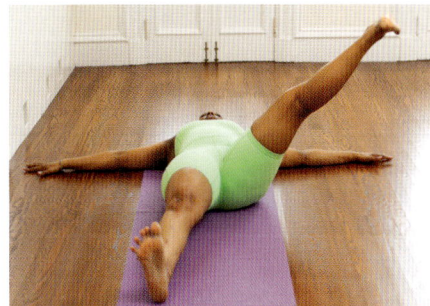

**FIGURE 2.141.** Alternate view.

repeat on the other side. It may take a few attempts to find the optimal range of motion where your hips, pelvis, and abdomen are stable. The emphasis should be on controlled movement rather than a big groin stretch. Think about your lower abdomen and pelvis as the "control center" that is directing and controlling the movement of your inclined leg, rather than your leg pulling your pelvis.

## VARIATIONS

WIDE HIPS OR BACK PAIN: Move your bottom leg farther out to the side so that your outer heel is more in line with your outer hip.

HIP PAIN IN YOUR BOTTOM LEG: Move your bottom heel wider and support it on a low block.

***Effects*** *This pose strengthens the medial buttock muscle, which in turn stabilizes the hip joint. It engages the TA and teaches how to stretch and move the legs while maintaining pelvic and abdominal stability.*

### 11. Jaṭhara Parivartānāsana with Knees Bent (Revolving Abdomen Pose)

Lie down with knees bent and belt your middle thighs so that the thighs come together firmly. Bring your knees as close into your chest as possible, keeping your sacrum and lumbar spine on the floor. Stretch your arms out to the sides in line with your shoulders, palms down. Maintaining a straight line from your tailbone to the center of your sternum to the crown of your head, slowly exhale and bring your knees to the right. Keep your knees tucked up toward your right armpit, with your feet, knees, and thighs pressing. Your bottom leg will want to slide away from the top leg. Draw back from your right outer thigh to your hip, moving your leg deeper into the socket. Your knees should not come all the way to the floor but should hover parallel to the floor. Maintain your knees turning to the right as you move your lower abdomen to the left, bringing the left side of your waist closer to the floor. Press down strongly through your left shoulder and

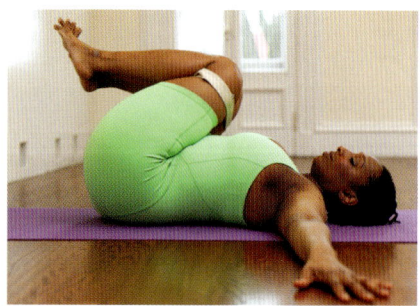

FIGURE 2.142. Jaṭhara Parivartānāsana, knees bent.

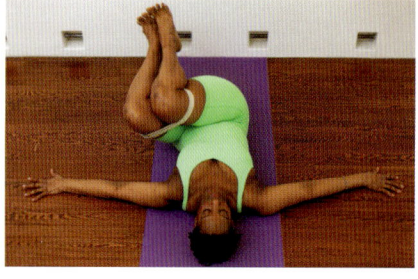

FIGURE 2.143. Alternate view.

reach out through your left arm. Stay for two or three breaths, then press your bottom leg up into your top leg to come up. Come back to center and repeat on the left side. This can be repeated several times with movement.

**Effects** *This pose tones the abdomen and engages the oblique muscles. It brings compactness to the outer thighs and hips. The twisting action generates a wringing action to the organs, which creates a detoxifying effect as fresh blood is brought to them.*

### 12. Śīrṣāsana with a Belt or a Band

Setup for Śīrṣāsana as in Week 5, pose 13. Have a belt looped about hips width, or a resistance band. Holding on to the loop with one toe, kick up into Śīrṣāsana and place the belt on your outer feet (the metatarsals) as in fig. 2.144. Alternately have a helper place the belt for you once you're up. Press out into the belt and feel the outer hips sucking in. The effects will be similar to those experienced in Sālamba Sarvāṅgāsana with the belt.

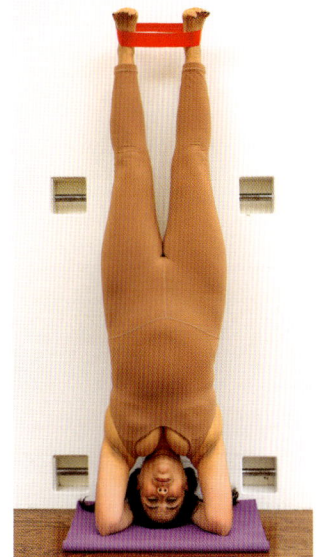

FIGURE 2.144. **Śīrṣāsana with a band.**

### 13. Sālamba Sarvāṅgāsana

See fig. 2.145 and Week 2 pose 6 for instructions.

### 14. Setubandha Sarvāṅgāsana (with Support)

See fig. 2.146 and Week 1 pose 7. for instructions.

### 15. Śavāsana

See fig. 2.147 and Week 1 pose 9 for instructions.

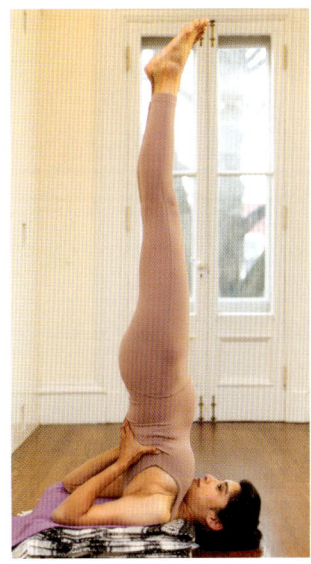

FIGURE 2.145. **Sālamba Sarvāṅgāsana.**

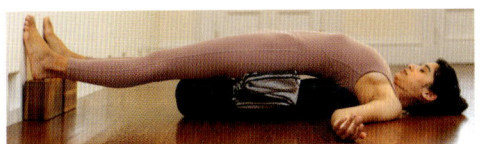

FIGURE 2.146. **Setubandha Sarvāṅgāsana.**

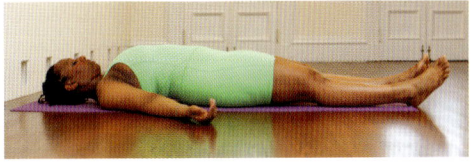

FIGURE 2.147. **Śavāsana.**

## WEEK 6 FULL SEQUENCE

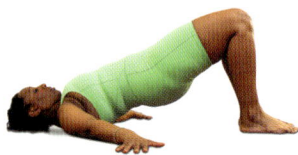 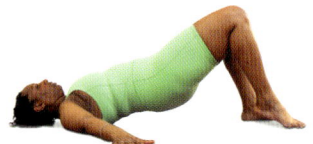 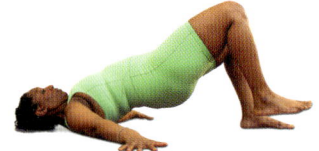

1. Ardha Setubandha, stage 1 (page 143)

Ardha Setubandha, stage 2 (page 145)

Ardha Setubandha, stage 3 (page 145)

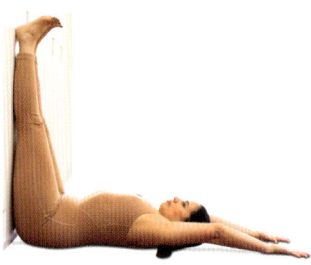 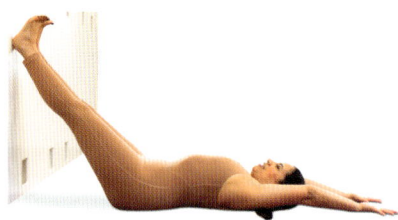

2. Ūrdhva Prasārita Pādāsana, 90 degrees (page 146)

3. Ūrdhva Prasārita Pādāsana, 60 degrees (page 148)

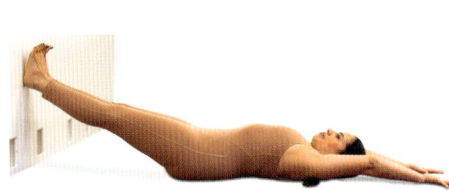 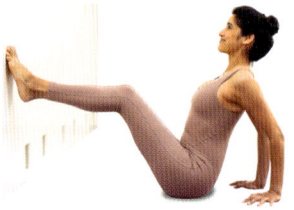

4. Ūrdhva Prasārita Pādāsana, 30 degrees (page 148)

5. Paripūrṇa Nāvāsana with bent knees, stage 1 (page 150)

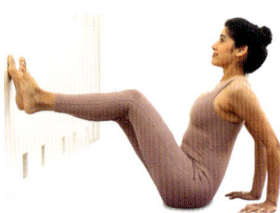 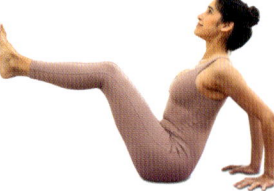 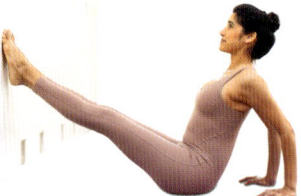

Paripūrṇa Nāvāsana with bent knees, stage 2 (page 150)

Paripūrṇa Nāvāsana with bent knees, stage 3 (page 150)

6. Paripūrṇa Nāvāsana with straight legs, stage 1 (page 151)

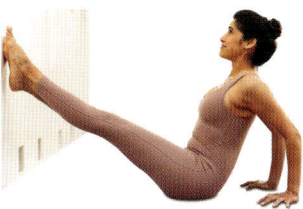

Paripūrṇa Nāvāsana with straight legs, stage 2 (page 151)

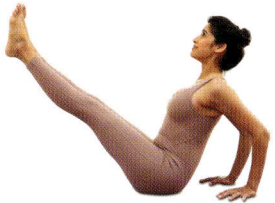

Paripūrṇa Nāvāsana with straight legs, stage 3 (page 152)

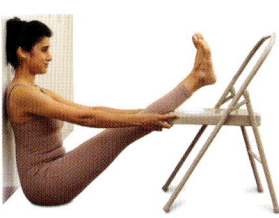

7.  Paripūrṇa Nāvāsana with a chair (page 152)

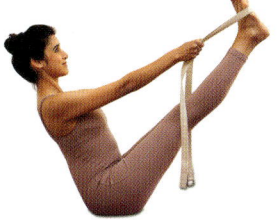

8.  Paripūrṇa Nāvāsana with a belt (page 153)

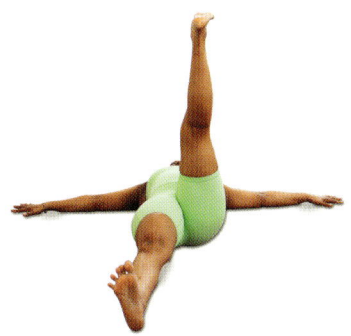

9.  Nirālamba Supta Pādāṅguṣṭhāsana I (page 154)

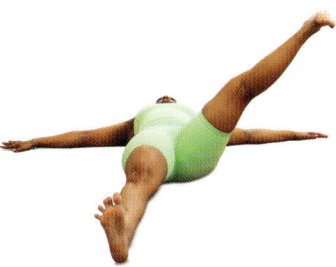

10.  Nirālamba Supta Pādāṅguṣṭhāsana II (page 155)

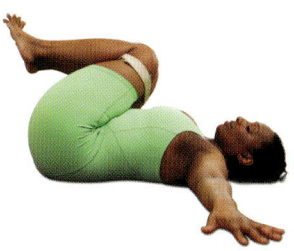

11.  Jaṭhara Parivartānāsana (page 156)

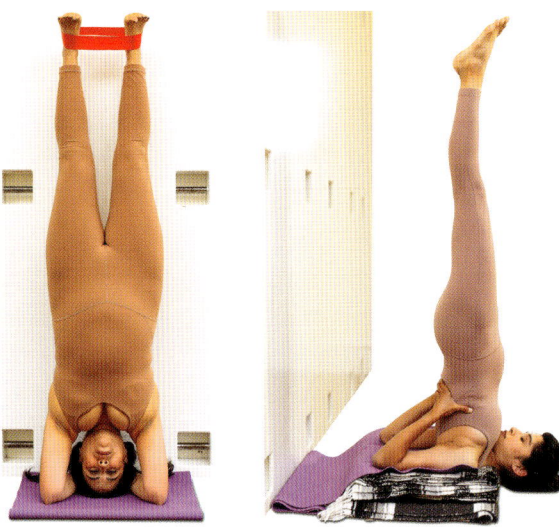

12. Śīrṣāsana
(page 157)

13. Sālamba
Sarvāṅgāsana (page 77)

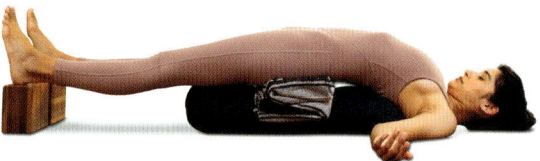

14. Setubandha Sarvāṅgāsana (page 63)

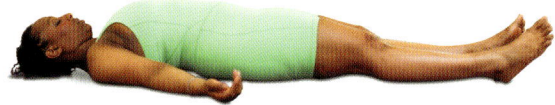

15. Śavāsana (page 65)

# Week 7
## AWAKENING *the* SPINE

Our final sequence brings together the knowledge from previous sequences and introduces twisting and backward-extending āsanas. After pregnancy and childbirth, some individuals find that these families of āsanas are the most difficult to return to. Oftentimes the work of carrying a baby to term followed by the hard work of feeding and caring for an infant without adequate rest can leave the spine feeling stiff and tired. Many new parents we've worked with over the years carry tension in the neck, shoulders, and wrists. Backward extensions, already a challenging family of āsanas, can be especially challenging after pregnancy as core and spinal strength and stability may be compromised. Even advanced practitioners may have to proceed slowly, maintaining control of the lower spine, abdomen, and pelvis to prevent injury.

The poses in this sequence focus on mobilizing stiffness and bringing energizing actions to the spine. Twisting poses bring mobility to the spine and nourishment to the organs. They have a detoxifying effect on the body. Backward extensions also mobilize the spine, especially when the focus is on the upper back and chest, as they are in this sequence. These poses can relieve sluggishness and bring vitality to the heart and lungs. Backbends may also benefit breast milk production for breastfeeding or chestfeeding individuals and relieve stiffness and soreness in the upper back and shoulders from nursing, co-sleeping, and carrying babies. Furthermore, many people with lower back pain benefit from increased mobility in the upper spine, which tends to be stiffer. Combined with intelligent pelvic floor and abdominal strengthening, those with lower back pain may find relief.

This sequence also introduces a number of variations of previous poses with slightly more elaborate setups or that require more experience and comfort with the props. Poses such as Adho Mukha Śvānāsana with high ropes, Nirālamba Sarvāṅgāsana, and Supta Koṇāsana can be practiced earlier during the postpartum recovery time, as soon as you are ready to begin inverting—around five or six weeks postpartum, but longer for Supta Koṇāsana, which requires greater groin spreading. They can be especially good for relieving pressure in the pelvic floor, correcting organ prolapse, and generally bringing the organs into their optimal positions. However, postpartum individuals should wait at least sixteen to twenty weeks before beginning twists and backward extensions. Those who are menstruating should avoid deep closed twists such as Marichyāsana III as well as the inversions in this sequence.

## Sequence of Āsanas: Week 7

### 1. Tāḍāsana with a Block

See fig. 2.148 and Week 4 pose 1 for instructions.

### 2. Ūrdhva Hastāsana

See fig. 2.149 and Week 4 pose 2 for instructions.

### 3. Ūrdhva Baddhanguliyāsana

See fig. 2.150 and Week 4 pose 3 for instructions.

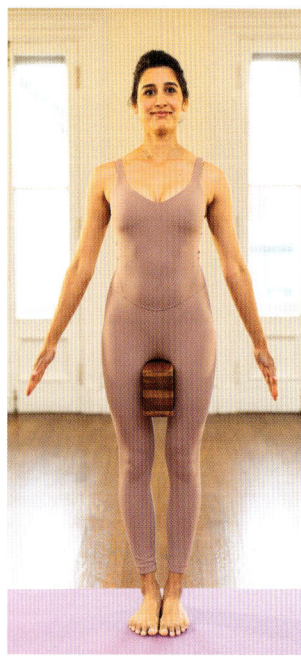
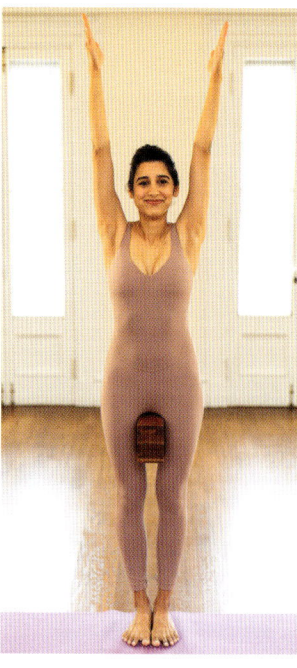
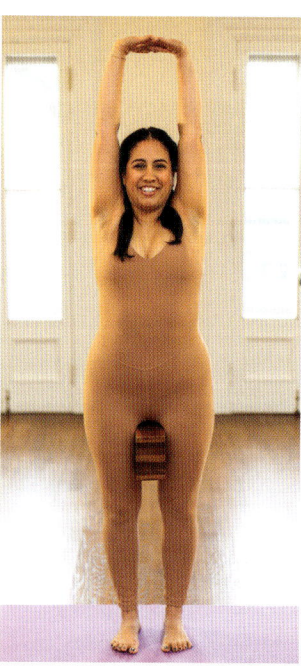

FIGURE 2.148. Tāḍāsana.

FIGURE 2.149. Ūrdhva Hastāsana.

FIGURE 2.150. Ūrdhva Baddhanguliyāsana.

### 4. GOMUKHĀSANA ARMS

See fig. 2.151 and Week 4 pose 4 for

### 5. PAŚCHIMA NAMASKĀRĀSANA

See fig. 2.152 and Week 4 pose 5 for instructions.

### 6. ADHO MUKHA ŚVĀNĀSANA

See Week 5, pose 3 (fig. 2.153) for instructions. Shown here is a version of the pose with a pair of high ropes, called "U-rope," for those who have access to ropes. The feet are supported on a Siṁhāsana box, and the hands are on blocks (fig. 2.154). This version of the pose is deeply restorative and brings tremendous length to the spine. It deepens the inverting quality of the pose with minimal effort and dramatically brings the pelvic organs toward the spine. It is particularly good for organ prolapse. This version could be introduced as soon as you feel ready for Adho Mukha Śvānāsana, as in Week 5.

### 7. PRASĀRITA PĀDOTTĀNĀSANA (WIDE-LEGGED INTENSE STRETCH POSE)

Stand in Tāḍāsana in the middle of the mat and step your legs five feet apart. Keep your toes pointing forward and press your outer heels down as you draw up from the inner arches to your inner knees. With your hands on your hips, lift the sides of your trunk and chest, bringing your shoulder blades down and in to make the

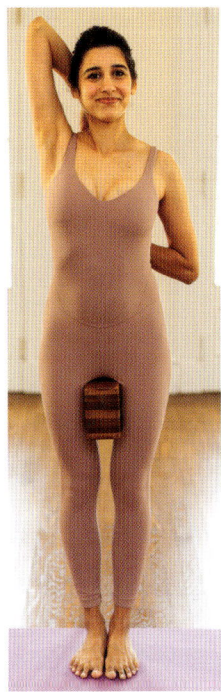
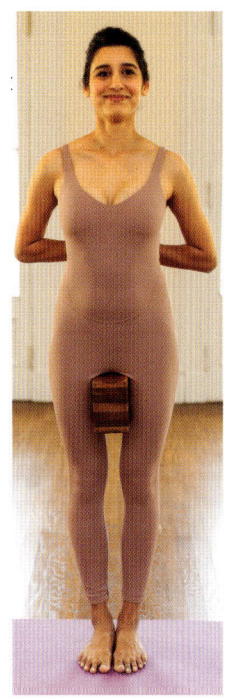

**FIGURE 2.151.**
**Gomukhāsana.**

**FIGURE 2.152.**
**Paśchima Namaskārāsana.**

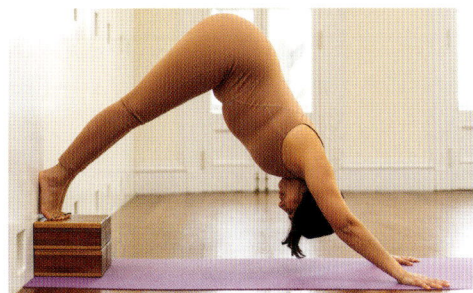

**FIGURE 2.153.**  **Adho Mukha Śvānāsana**

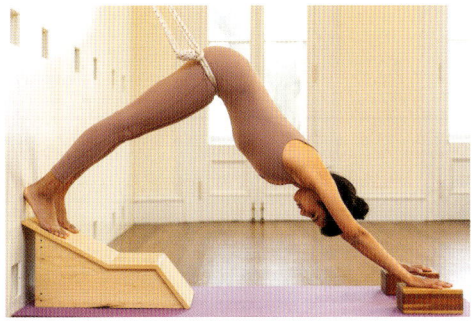

**FIGURE 2.154.**  **Adho Mukha Śvānāsana elevated with ropes.**

thoracic spine concave. Keeping your chest open, fold forward from your hips, while strongly lifting the backs of your thighs and spreading your buttocks. Place your hands on the floor, directly under your shoulders, and with your arms straight. If your hands do not reach the floor, support them on bricks (fig. 2.155). Press your palms into the floor and stretch the sides of your waist and chest forward as you move the roots of your thighs back. This is the concave spine stage of the pose (fig. 2.156). Beginners or those with a lot of stiffness can practice this stage only for some time until there is enough freedom to proceed further.

From here, continue to lift the backs of your thighs as you walk your hands back toward your feet and lengthen the sides of your trunk down, the crown of your head resting on the floor or on a block (fig. 2.157). Take care that your spine doesn't round as your head comes down. Walk your hands as far back in line with your feet as possible, fingers pointing forward, and gently press your hands down to lift your shoulders away from your ears. Learn to release the buttock flesh and lumbar spine toward your head to bring more weight to your head. Stay for two or three breaths. To come out, walk your hands forward, grip your outer hips, and raise your trunk up.

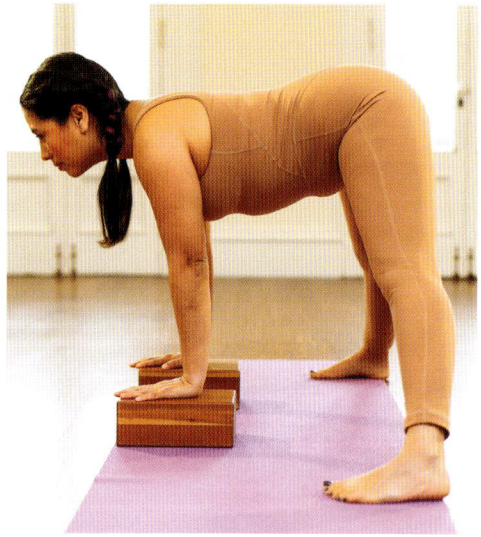

FIGURE 2.155. **Prasārita Pādottānāsana with concave spine.**

## VARIATIONS

HIP AND PELVIC INSTABILITY: Start with your feet closer together,

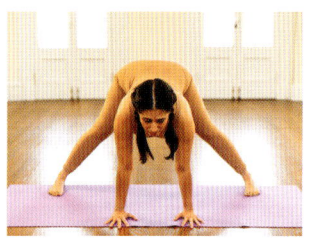

FIGURE 2.156. **Alternate view.**

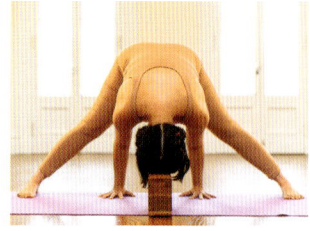

FIGURE 2.157. **Head down**

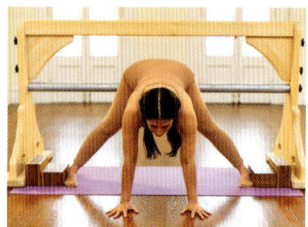

FIGURE 2.158. **Feet blocked in a trestle**

and place your hands on a higher support, like two blocks or a chair. Practice coming in and out of the pose slowly from this higher support, working on evenly drawing your outer hips in and back, and moving the femur bones toward each other and deeper into the sockets. The movement should be even and smooth. Once the movement is controlled, then gradually lower the height of your hands and head. Alternatively, block the outer edges of your feet in, using a wide hallway or trestle (fig. 2.158). Blocks can be inserted to create the correct width of the legs. Press your outer feet into the blocks or walls to further draw the femurs into the sockets, creating stability.

**Effects** *This pose stretches and strengthens the legs and spine. It widens and spreads the pelvic floor. The final stage of this pose inverts the pelvis and is good for organ prolapse as well as preparing you for inversions like Śīrṣāsana. It rests and quiets the brain.*

### 8. Pārśvottānāsana

Follow instructions for Pārśvottānāsana from Week 2, pose 5. Then proceed by bringing your hands down to the floor or blocks. Maintain the length of your spine by strongly lengthening the sides of your waist forward and bringing your back ribs and shoulder blades into your body (fig. 2.159). From here, you can progress by bending your elbows and lengthening the front of your torso down your leg, eventually bringing your forehead to your shin (fig. 2.160).

**Effects** *This pose lengthens, stretches, and strengthens the spine and legs.*

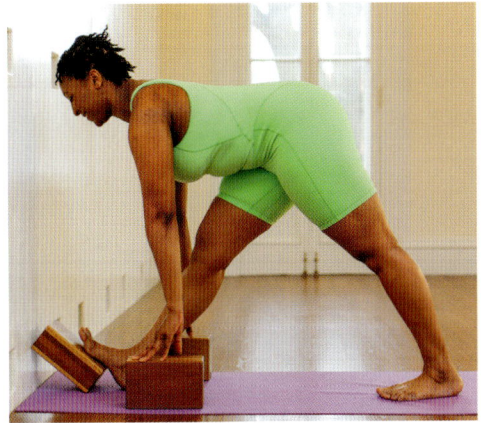

**FIGURE 2.159.** Pārśvottānāsana with concave spine.

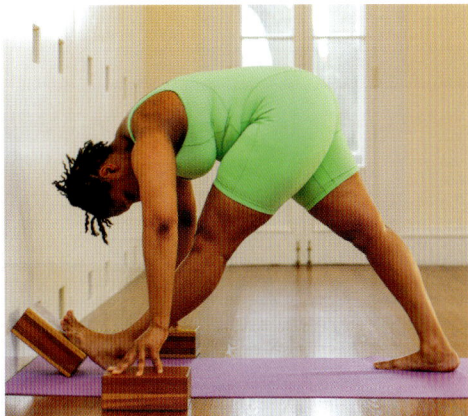

**FIGURE 2.160.** Full pose

## 9. Parivṛtta Trikoṇāsana (Revolved Triangle Pose)

Stand in Tāḍāsana in the middle of the mat and step your feet four to four and a half feet apart, with a block placed on its highest height on the right side of the mat. With your hands on your hips, turn your right leg out 90 degrees, turn your left foot in, and revolve your torso to face your right leg. Keep your feet in line with each other. As you press your back outer heel down, revolve the back of your back thigh from inside out. Draw your outer hips in and lift the sides of your waist up. Stretch your arms out to the sides in a T-shape, and reaching forward with your left arm, revolve your whole torso to the right, placing your left hand down on the block on the outside of your right foot. Bring your right arm onto your hip. Keeping your feet and hips stable, turn your abdomen, waist, and chest from left to right. Roll your right shoulder back. Move your head back and open your chest so there is a straight line from your back heel to the center of your pelvis to the crown of your head. Now reach your arms strongly away from each other as you spread your chest and turn it up toward the ceiling. Keep your head in line with your spine and look forward, and then up, if your neck allows. Take two or three quiet breaths. To come out, press your back heel and reach with your top arm to come up. Turn your feet parallel and step your legs together. Repeat on the opposite side.

### VARIATIONS

STIFF LEGS AND SPINE OR BACKACHE: Place the block on the inside of your front foot and step your feet slightly away from your midline. Beginners or those returning to this pose after some time may also benefit from practicing this way until more strength and stability come in the legs. You may also place your bottom hand on a higher support and your top hand on a trestle, window ledge, or counter and press down to help lift and turn your abdomen and chest.

SHOULDER PAIN, TIGHT SHOULDERS OR SPINE: Keep your top hand on your waist and

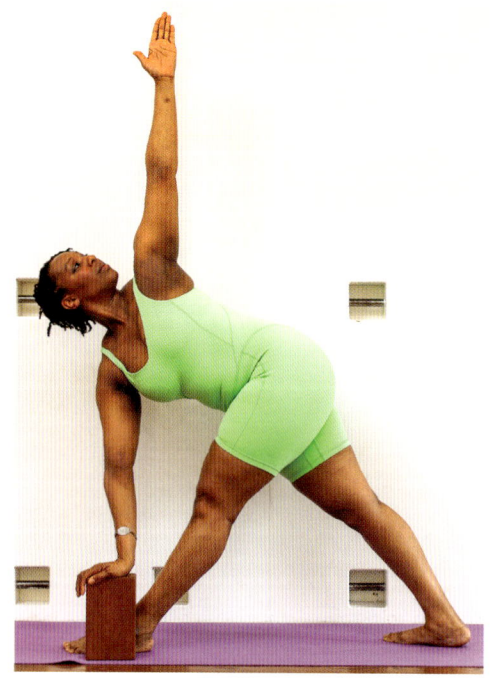

FIGURE 2.161. Parivṛtta Trikoṇāsana.

use your bent elbow to turn better, bringing your shoulder blades deeper against your back ribs to help open the thoracic spine.

**Effects** *Creates a "wringing" effect on the spine, spinal muscles, and organs. Aids in circulation to these areas, helping tonify the pelvic and abdominal organs, and aiding in digestion.*

### 10. Parivṛtta Vīrabhadrāsana I (Revolved Warrior I Pose)

Position a mat lengthwise at the wall. With your right hip near the wall, step your right foot forward and your left foot back, four to four and a half feet apart. Turn your back toes out slightly but keep your back thigh and hip revolving forward. Bend your front knee, moving your right buttock toward your right knee. Keep your tailbone moving in and the front of your pelvis lifting. You are now in Vīrabhadrāsana I, with the wall to your right. Keeping your chest lifted, revolve your abdomen, waist, and chest toward the wall. Bend your elbows and place your fingertips at the wall. Pull down with your fingertips to lift the front of your pelvis and abdomen up. Bring your shoulder blades onto your back ribs and press more with your right hand to turn the thoracic spine more. Stay for two or three breaths and then release and repeat on the other side. At first you may not be able to bend your knee very far, and turning will feel difficult. The priority

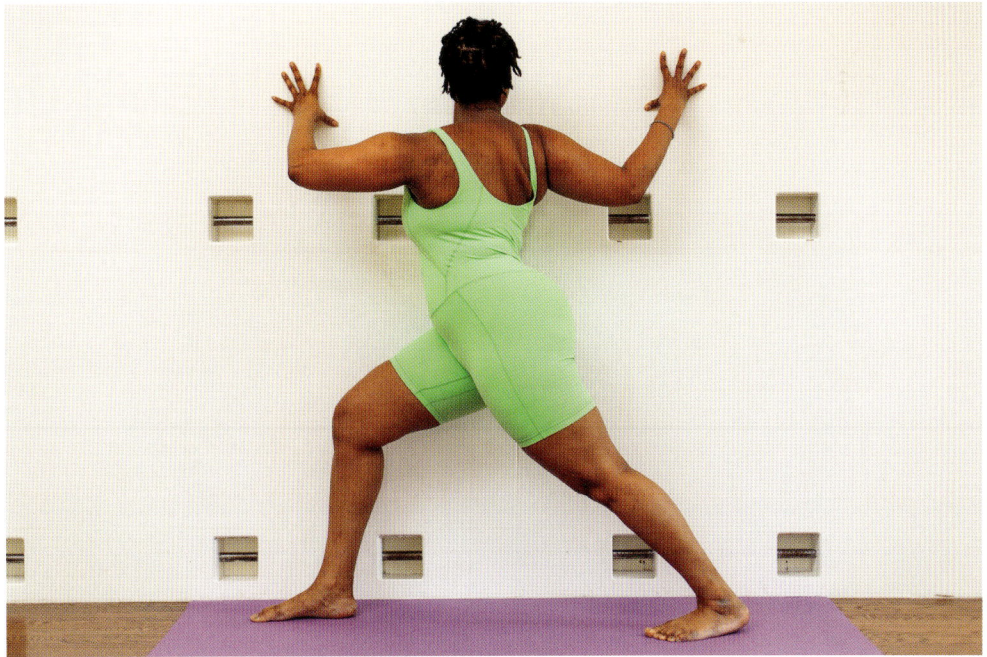

FIGURE 2.162.  **Parivṛtta Vīrabhadrāsana I.**

should be to keep the lifting actions of your pelvis and the pelvic organs rather than bending your knee deeply.

## VARIATIONS

For better support, use a trestle, window ledge, or countertop to press your hands down. This will give you better lifting actions in your abdomen and pelvis.

*Effects Relieves tension and stiffness in the lower spine and thoracic spine. Introduces deeper abdominal turning than Pariv r̥tta Trikoṇāsana and teaches the correct lifting action needed before proceeding to stronger twists.*

### 11. Śīrṣāsana

See fig. 2.163 and Week 5 pose 13 for instructions.

### 12. Dwipāda Viparīta Daṇḍāsana (Two-Legged Inverted Staff Pose)

Place a chair near a wall with the backrest facing the wall. Place a twice-folded sticky mat on the seat of a chair, two blocks against the wall, and a bolster in front of the chair. Sit through the chair facing the wall, with your knees bent. If you do not have a backless chair, you can use a regular chair and sit sideways. Hold the sides of the chair and, lifting your chest, lie back with your shoulder blades on the edge of the chair. Slide your hands down the backrest of the chair, pull down, and draw your shoulder blades away from your ears and strongly onto the back ribs to coil your chest more over the edge of the chair. Coil off the chair more and place the crown of your head on the bolster. If your head doesn't easily

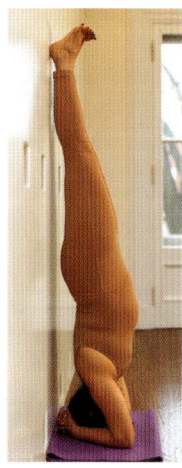

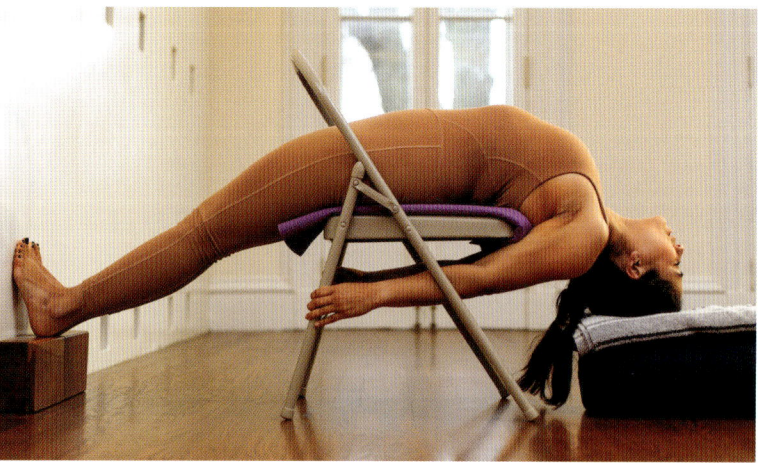

**FIGURE 2.163.** Śīrṣāsana.

**FIGURE 2.164.** Dwipāda Viparīta Daṇḍāsana.

reach, come up and add a blanket on top of the bolster, rather than pushing your spine more off the chair. The aim is to keep the fulcrum of the backbend in the upper armpit chest rather than toward the lumbar spine. Especially for postpartum individuals, too much lower thoracic and lumbar opening can be too intense or even dangerous as there is not enough abdominal stability to counter the increased pressure on the lumbar spine and abdominal and pelvic organs. As your chest coils more, you can attempt to bring your arms under the seat of the chair, holding the back legs of the chair for increased freedom in your chest and shoulders. Once the position of your head and chest is in place, straighten your legs one at a time toward the wall, heels supported up on the blocks, legs together (fig. 2.164). At first, it may be difficult to bring the legs absolutely together; in this case, keep them hips width apart. Beginners can stay for thirty to sixty seconds. Over time you can gradually build up to several minutes, which will increase the positive benefits of the pose. To come up, bend your knees and return your feet to the floor, hold the sides of your chair, and keeping the coil of the chest, lift your chest up all in one action. Sit straight and take a few breaths to recover before coming out of the chair.

## VARIATIONS

BACKACHE: Support your feet higher on blocks or a stool with your feet hips width apart. A belt can be placed around your upper thighs or outer hips for more pelvic and lumbar stability.

NECK PAIN: Support your head with extra blankets so the back of your head is more parallel to the floor, eyes facing up toward the ceiling.

LOWER BACK PAIN: Place a folded blanket under your tailbone to provide extra lift and facilitate spreading of the lower back and abdomen. This pose can also be practiced with the "cone" adjustment (see Week 2, pose 8).

**Effects** *This pose strongly opens the chest and brings energy and mobility to the upper spine. It energizes the heart and lungs and can help with depression, sluggish thyroid, and other hormonal imbalances. It also promotes milk production in lactating people and can bring relief to pain in the shoulders and upper back from breastfeeding or chestfeeding, co-sleeping, and carrying babies.*

### 13. Pūrvottānāsana with Support (Intense Front-Stretch Pose)

Stand with your back to the trestle, feet slightly wider than your hips. Move your hands back onto the trestle, hands wide, then bending your knees, lower your upper back and shoulder blades onto the trestle. Hold the back of your head in

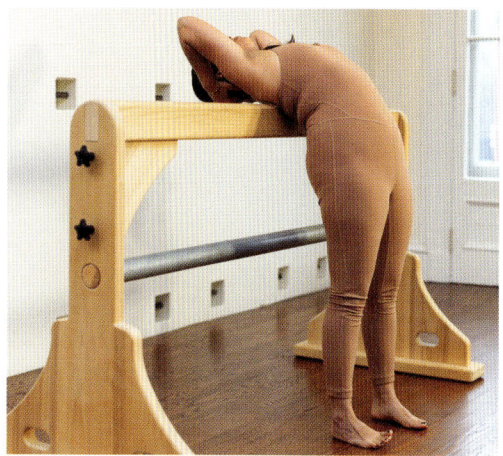

FIGURE 2.165. **Pūrvottānāsana with trestle.**

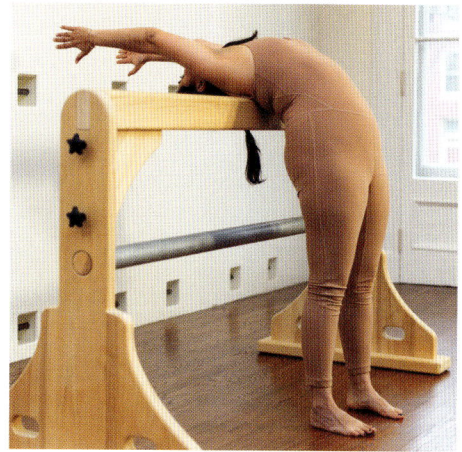

FIGURE 2.166. **Arms overhead.**

your hands and coil your upper back over the top of the trestle, using your hands to support the whole weight of your head (fig. 2.165). Press your inner heels and inner ball mounds of your feet down strongly, and broaden the backs of your thighs, making sure your feet, knees, and thighs do not splay outward. Keep your tailbone moving in and lift strongly through your lumbar spine and back ribs. Draw your outer arms in and aim your elbows back to deepen the coiling action. If your lower back feels tense, walk your feet out slightly, or raise your heels up, lengthening your buttocks away from the lumbar spine toward the backs of your knees. To deepen the pose, walk your feet in slightly and straighten your legs, pressing the shinbones back as you lift from the backs of your thighs upward. Move your arms overhead for an even deeper opening of the chest and shoulders (fig. 2.166). Stay for three to five breaths, keeping your abdomen soft and lengthened. To come out, bend your knees, raise your head, and press your palms down on the trestle to lift your chest up, coming back to standing. This can be repeated several times, staying for more cycles of breath according to your capacity.

## VARIATIONS

For those who don't have access to a trestle, this pose can be practiced over the back of a couch, high banister or railing, or any other sturdy high support.

*Effects* *This pose strongly opens the chest and brings energy and mobility to the upper spine. It energizes the heart and lungs and can help with depression, sluggish thyroid, and other hormonal imbalances. It also promotes milk production in lactating people and can bring relief to pain in the shoulders and upper back from breastfeeding or chestfeeding, co-sleeping, and carrying babies.*

### 14. BHARADVĀJĀSANA I

Sit in Daṇḍāsana on two folded blankets. Bend your knees to the left so that your left foot rests on top of the right arch with your toes pointing back, as in Vīrāsana. Your right (bottom) toes should point to the side. Shift your weight so that only your right buttock is supported on the blanket, with your left buttock off. Keep your knees together, pointing forward. Check to see that your hips are even by moving your left buttock farther down. Stretch your arms and the sides of your waist up and turn to the right, placing your left hand on your right outer knee, and your right hand as far back on the blanket toward your left buttock as possible. Lift the sides of your waist up, and on an exhalation, turn your abdomen, ribs, and chest from left to right. Roll your right shoulder back and pin your right shoulder blade in to open the chest more. Keep your head and neck in line with the sternum, your eyes and face quiet. Take two or three breaths, then release and repeat on the other side. This pose can be repeated several times, especially for those with stiffness in the ankles, knees, hips, spine, and shoulders.

#### VARIATIONS

KNEE, HIP, OR LOWER BACK PAIN: Sit in a chair as in the standing and seated āsanas in Week 4.

***Effects*** *This pose brings a wringing effect to the organs and spine, improving circulation and digestion. It brings mobility to the knees, hips, shoulders, and upper back. It also relieves backache, especially after backward extensions.*

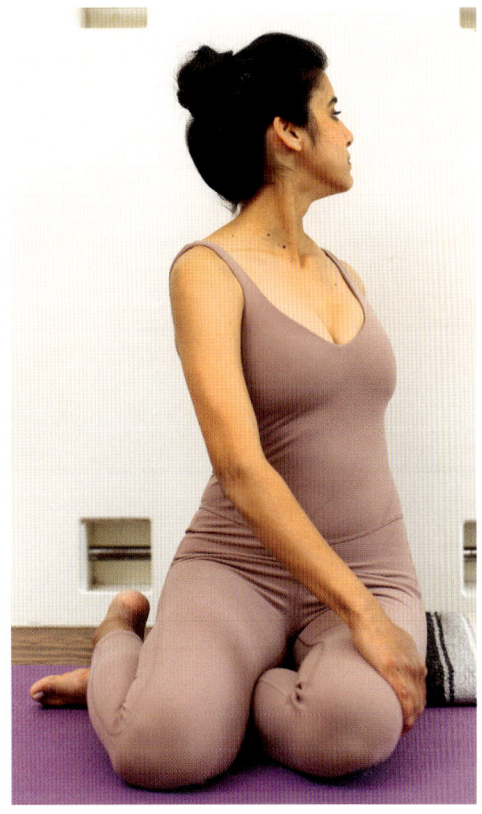

FIGURE 2.167. **Bharadvājāsana I.**

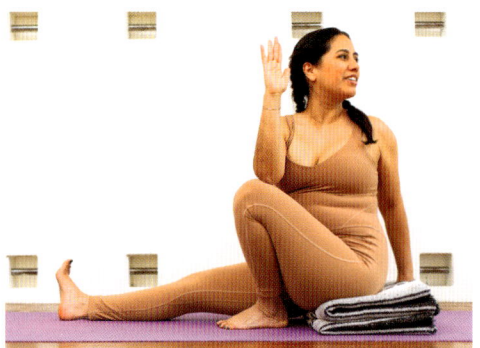

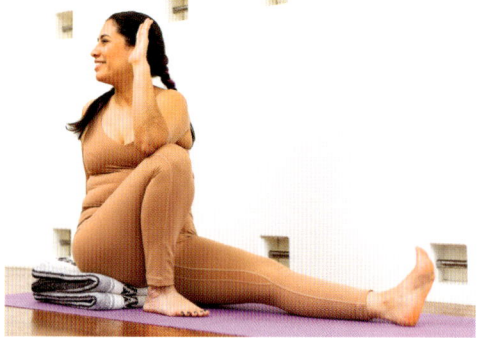

FIGURE 2.168. **Marichyāsana III.**       FIGURE 2.169. **Alternate view.**

## 15. Marichyāsana III (Sage Marichi's Twist Pose)

Sit in Daṇḍāsana on two folded blankets. Bend your right knee in toward your chest, placing your heel near the buttock bone with your toes pointing forward. Lift your arms up, stretching the sides of your trunk upward, and with an exhalation, turn to the right. Bend your left arm and hook your left elbow on the outside of your right knee (fig. 2.169). Reach your right hand as far back on the blanket toward your left buttock as possible. Use your back hand to press and lift the spine upward as you turn your abdomen, waist, and chest from left to right. Bring more of your left outer elbow to your right outer knee and press into the knee to bring your left back ribs and kidney area deeper into the body. Bring your shoulder blades down your back as you lift and spread the collarbones, broadening your top chest. Keep your head in line with your tailbone, eyes forward and quiet. Take two or three breaths, then release and repeat on the other side (fig. 2.168). This pose can be repeated several times, especially for those with stiffness in the ankles, knees, hips, spine, and shoulders.

*Effects This pose deeply rotates the lower spine, bringing mobility and a massaging action to the rib cage and organs. It improves circulation and digestion, and the squeezing effect on the kidneys and adrenals may help support the endocrine system.*

## 16. Sālamba Sarvāṅgāsana Supported on a Chair

Read through the instructions for poses 16 to 18, as you will be using the same setup to move from Sālamba Sarvāṅgāsana to Nirālamba Sarvāṅgāsana and Supta Koṇāsana. Place a sticky mat, folded in quarters, on the seat of a chair with the seat facing the wall about two feet away from it. Place a bolster horizontally on the floor between the chair and the wall, leaving a gap of six to eight inches between the bolster and the wall. If you have sensitivity when resting the back of your head on the floor, a thin blanket can be placed on the floor between the bolster and the wall. Sit on the chair with your back toward the wall and your knees hooked over the top of the chair. Holding the sides of the chair, lift your spine and chest up (fig. 2.170), and lie back so that the tops of your shoulders come down to the bolster, and your head rests on the floor, with your neck supported by the bolster. There should be a small gap between the top of your head and the wall—at no point should your head touch the wall. If you are shorter, you may need to unhook your legs to come down all the way onto the bolster. Now your sacrum should be resting on the seat of the chair, holding the weight of the pose. Move your hands just below the joint of the chair, bend your elbows, and turn your arms strongly from inside out. Lift your back ribs up, bringing your shoulder blades into the body to dome your chest. Keeping your sacrum on the chair, stretch your legs straight, resting on the upper backrest of the chair (fig. 2.171). After a few breaths here, stretch your legs vertically, keeping your legs firmly pressing together (fig. 2.172). Keep your back ribs lifting actively so that your rib cage lengthens away from your pelvis. Keep your abdomen soft and your breath quiet. Rest the back of your head on the floor, soften your throat, and quiet your eyes. Stay for two or three minutes or to your capacity. At this stage, you can come down or proceed to pose 17, Nirālamba Sarvāṅgāsana. To come down, bend your knees, place your feet on the seat of the chair, and push the chair away from the wall, slowly sliding your head up onto the bolster and your buttocks down to the floor.

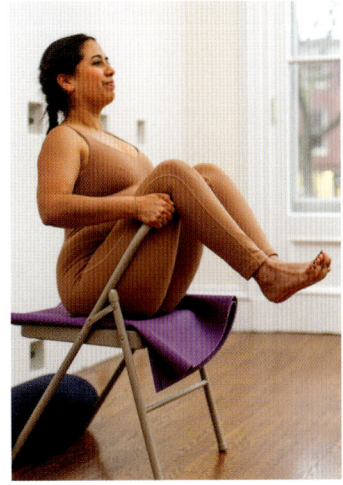

FIGURE 2.170. **Getting into Sālamba Sarvāṅgāsana.**

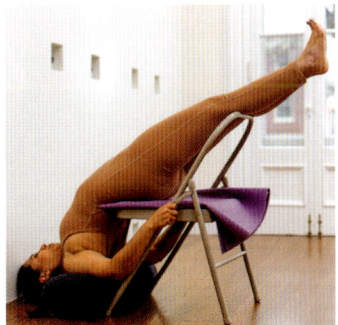

FIGURE 2.171. **Legs resting.**

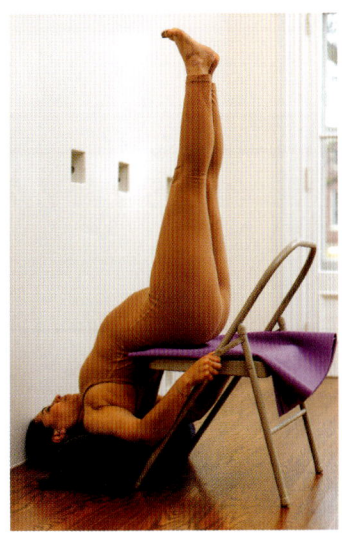

FIGURE 2.172. **Legs vertical.**

## VARIATIONS

LOWER BACK PAIN: Raise the height of the chair with a folded blanket so your pelvis is higher.

FATIGUE AND DEEPER ABDOMINAL RELAXATION: Have a helper place a bolster vertically between the backs of your legs and the backrest of the chair, then rest your legs on the bolster. Two bolsters may be needed to accommodate the width of your hips and legs.

**Effects** *This pose has similar effects to Sālamba Sarvāṅgāsana and Viparīta Karaṇī, however here the chest gets a bigger opening, stretching the heart, lungs, and diaphragm. The abdominal cavity and its contents are gently stretched toward the chest while the pelvic organs rest toward the sacrum, and these areas get fresh blood flow. Additionally, because of the action of jālandhara bandha (chin lock), the thyroid gets stimulated, making this pose helpful for balancing the endocrine and hormonal system. It is deeply quieting and leaves you feeling refreshed in body and mind.*

### 17. NIRĀLAMBA SARVĀṄGĀSANA (UNSUPPORTED ALL-LIMBED POSE OR SHOULDER STAND)

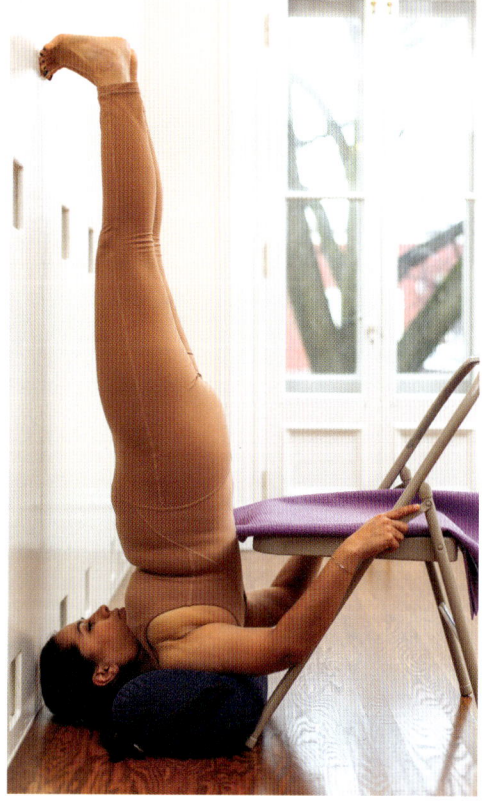

From pose 16, keep holding the outside of the chair, and with a swinging motion raise your feet, legs, and pelvis away from the chair, placing your feet on the wall. Keeping your toes tucked, walk your feet farther up the wall to lift your buttocks strongly so that your pelvis is directly above your shoulders. If you are new to practicing this pose, or if you are tight in the shoulders, you may want to keep your hands on the chair to encourage the turning of your upper arms and to create steadiness. If you have more experience, you can rest your arms on the floor with your elbows bent, hands near your ears. Take care to keep the bolster well under your

FIGURE 2.173. **Nirālamba Sarvāṅgāsana.**

shoulders and neck, and keep your shoulder blades tucked in so that the weight of the pose comes more to the top of your shoulders. Keep reaching your inner legs and buttocks up strongly so that your spine becomes light. Relax your throat and let your chin move toward your chest into a deep jālandhara bandha. Stay for two or three minutes or to your capacity. At this stage, you can come out or continue to pose 18, Supta Koṇāsana. To come out, hold the chair and bring your pelvis back onto the seat of the chair, then come out as described in pose 16.

## VARIATIONS

DEEPER LEG WORK: Experienced students can place a block high up between the thighs and a belt around, or just under, the block at the middle thigh. This creates a similar action as in the standing poses, Sālamba Sarvāṅgāsana, and Śīrṣāsana with the block.

***Effects*** *This pose has similar effects to Sālamba Sarvāṅgāsana, however here the back body feels long and light, and more softness comes to the organs as they rest backward toward the spine. This version of Sarvāṅgāsana teaches the lift of the buttocks and the firmness of the back legs and is good for those who may be struggling with these areas in Sālamba Sarvāṅgāsana. Practitioners who have experienced a cesarean section have reported that this pose feels soothing to the abdomen. Additionally, the action of jālandhara bandha (chin lock) is at a maximum, stimulating and balancing the endocrine and hormonal system. This pose brings quietness to the mind and a deep feeling of relaxation.*

### 18. Supta Koṇāsana (Supine Wide-Angle Pose)

From pose 17, stretch your legs wide apart, bringing the inner edges of your feet onto the wall, your toes pointing downward. If your inner legs feel too tight to move them wide apart, come back to pose 16 with your knees bent and your feet on the top of the chair, and using your hands against the wall, push the whole setup and your body a few more inches away from the wall, making sure you are stable and not slipping off your props. Come back into the pose and see if you have more room to stretch your legs wide. Stretch from your inner thighs to your inner heels, pressing the

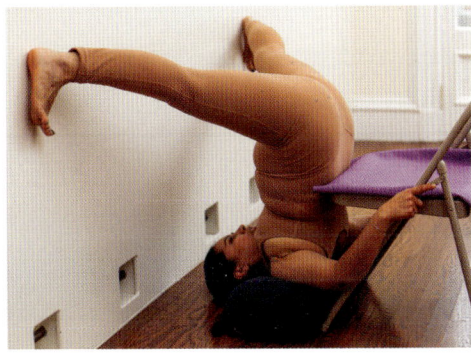

**FIGURE 2.174.  Supta Koṇāsana**

inner heels into the wall as you pull back from the outer edges of your feet toward the hip joints. Suck your outer thighs in toward the hip joints. Lift from your outer hips and back ribs so the spine stays long and the organs are uplifted. Relax your throat and soften your eyes, mouth, and face, breathing quietly for two or three minutes or to your capacity. To come out, raise your legs back up to pose 17, then return to the chair and come out as described in pose 16.

**Effects** *This pose continues the work of Nirālamba Sarvāṅgāsana. Here, the spreading of the legs creates more space in the pelvis, while the pelvic organs are naturally drawn inward, making this pose excellent for reducing pelvic organ prolapse and relieving any associated heaviness.*

### 19. Viparīta Karaṇī

Place a blanket, folded in half lengthwise, on top of a bolster and place them about three inches from the wall, running lengthwise. Sit sideways on the bolster, lean sideways toward the floor, and keeping your buttocks touching the wall, swing your legs up the wall, and lie back. Use your hands on the floor overhead to push your buttocks up against the wall so the whole back of your leg is in contact with the wall. The bolster and blanket should support your lumbar spine and the top of your sacrum, and the buttock bones should hang slightly off the edge of the bolster between the bolster and the wall. This provides a soothing effect to the lower back, especially after twisting. Stretch your legs up the wall with your legs together. You can tie a belt around your thighs to keep them in place without effort. Keep your shoulder blades moving down your back, and your top chest open. Rest with your palms up. Soften and spread your abdomen as you simultaneously spread the lumbar spinal muscles laterally. Go back to the breathing that was first presented in Week 1, observing how the pelvic floor and diaphragm soften and spread on the inhalation and gently contract on the exhalation. Spread your eyes and the skin of your face, resting your face completely. Stay for three to five minutes.

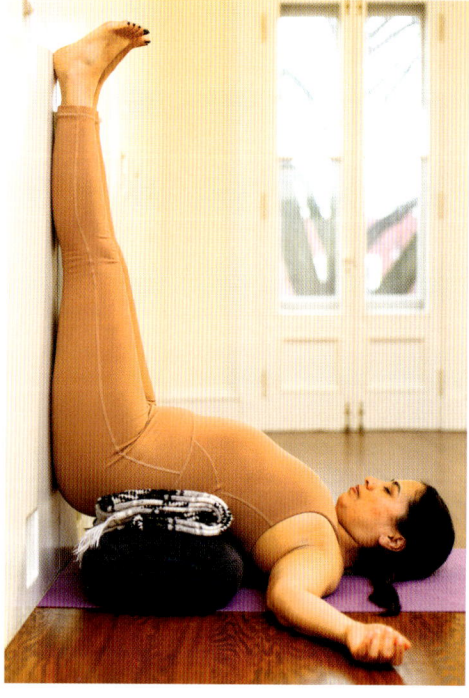

FIGURE 2.175.  **Viparīta Karaṇī.**

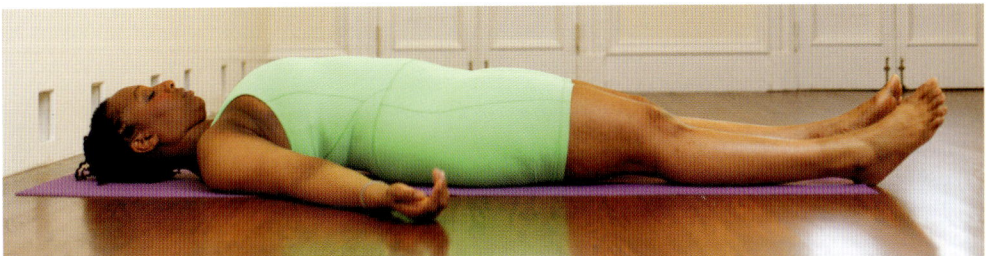

**FIGURE 2.176.** Śavāsana

**Effects** *This inversion releases tension in the lumbar spine, hips, and abdomen. It creates softening in the groins and abdomen and teaches the relaxation of the pelvic floor muscles. It also relieves fatigue, quiets the mind, and brings serenity to the whole nervous system.*

## 20. Śavāsana

See fig. 2.176 and Week 1 pose 9. for instructions.

### WEEK 7 FULL SEQUENCE

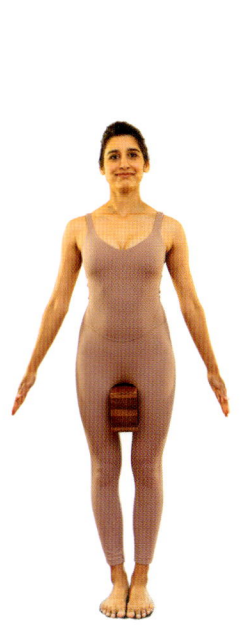

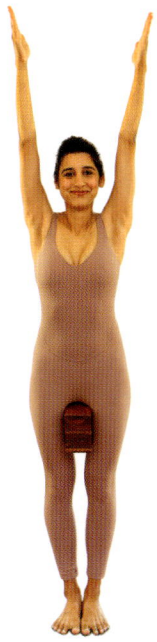

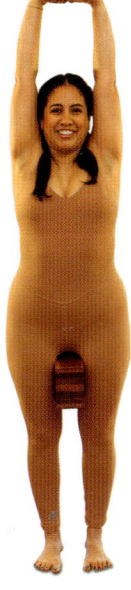

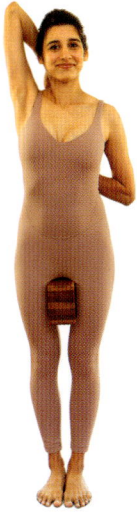

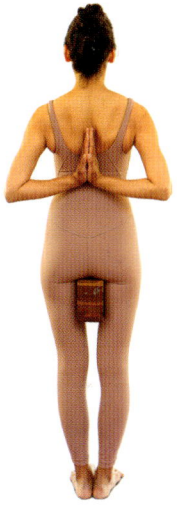

1. Tāḍāsana (page 102)

2. Ūrdhva Hastāsana (page 103)

3. Ūrdhva Baddhanguliyāsana (page 104)

4. Gomukhāsana arms (page 105)

5. Paśchima Namaskārāsana (page 106)

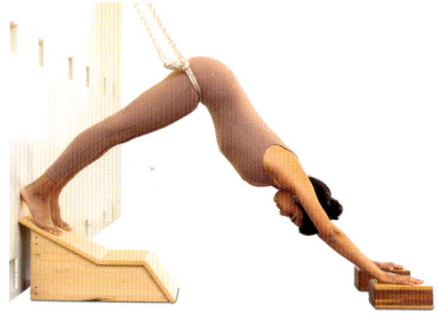

6. Adho Mukha Śvānāsana (page 163)

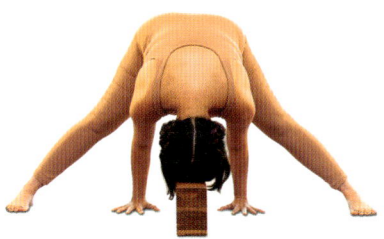

7. Prasārita Pādottānāsana (page 163)

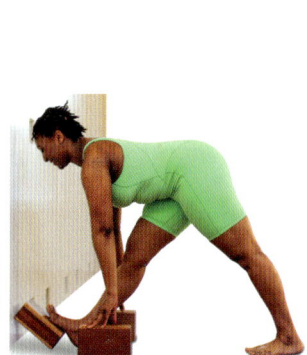

8. Pārśvottānāsana (page 165)

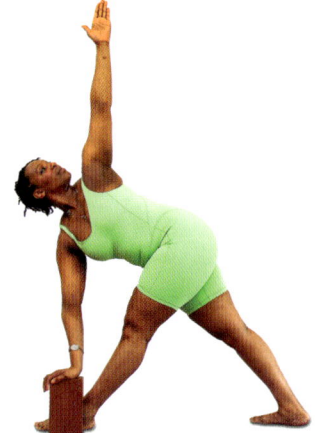

9. Parivṛtta Trikoṇāsana (page 166)

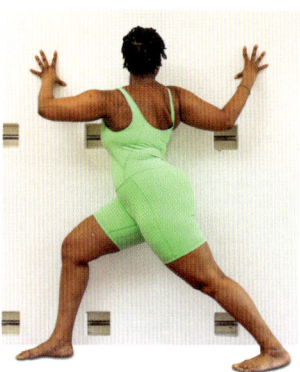

10. Parivṛtta Vīrabha-drāsana I (page 167)

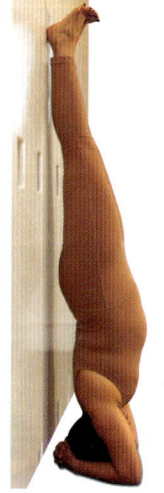

11. Śīrṣāsana (page 134)

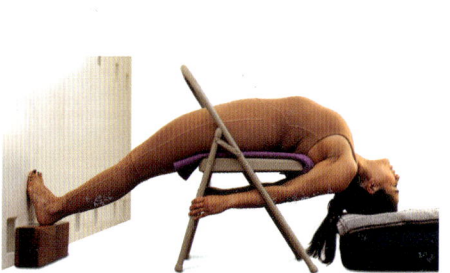

12. Dwipāda Viparīta Daṇḍāsana (page 168)

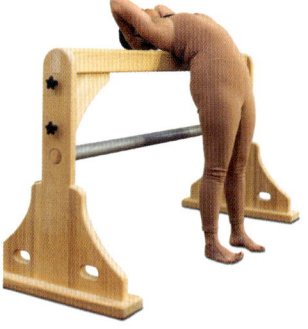

13. Pūrvottānāsana (page 169)

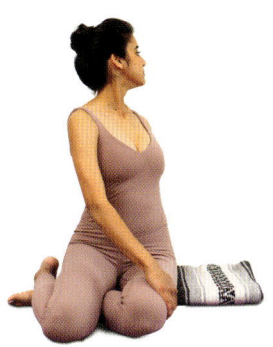

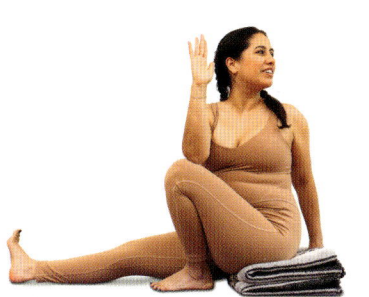

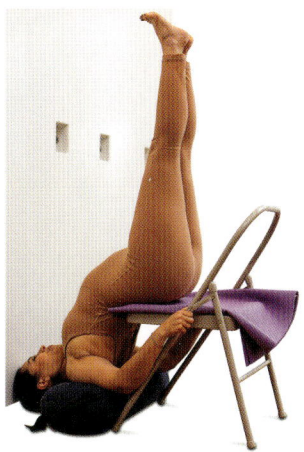

14. **Bharadvājāsana I** (page 171)

15. **Marichyāsana III** (page 172)

16. **Sālamba Sarvāṅgāsana on a chair** (page 172)

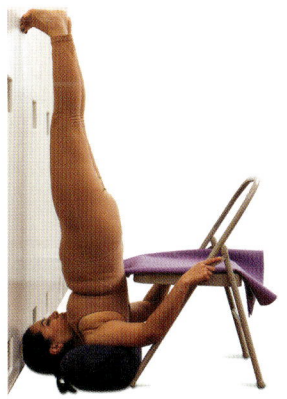

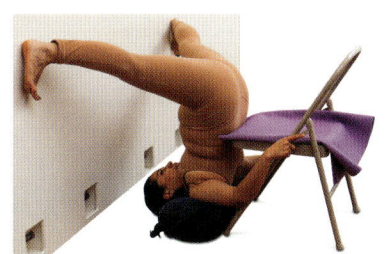

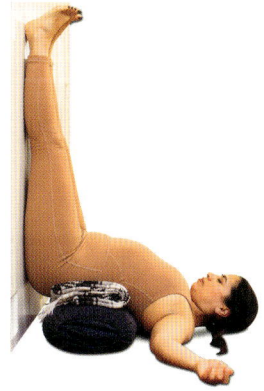

17. **Nirālamba Sarvāṅgāsana** (page 174)

18. **Supta Koṇāsana** (page 175)

19. **Viparīta Karaṇī** (page 176)

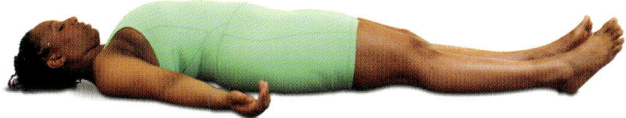

20. **Śavāsana** (page 65)

# SPECIAL TOPICS

In the following chapter, you will find an in-depth discussion of a variety of symptoms and conditions that we have found to be quite common in students who are postpartum or who are seeking help with their pelvic floor. We have found that practicing āsana and prāṇāyāma can be a great aid and tool, empowering students and complementing other modes of treatment. Yoga alone may not be enough to treat more serious symptoms, but it *can* help you gain a heightened awareness of the issue, provide anatomical and descriptive language to discuss it, and develop sensitivity to how movements or situations affect your symptoms, which can be greatly beneficial when seeking help from multiple practitioners. In other words, the approach to treatment may need to be multifaceted, and the more you can feel and communicate about your concerns, the better. The recommendations given here are not meant to replace medical help, and we encourage you to seek the advice of a pelvic floor specialist or trained pelvic health care provider, especially if symptoms are severe.

In this chapter we first offer relevant clinical information from the perspective of a pelvic health physical therapist that we think is helpful for the practicing student to know, followed by guidelines for how to approach your practice of āsana and prāṇāyāma from the perspective of Iyengar yoga. The following sections are not exhaustive, nor are they one-size-fits-all, and like elsewhere in this book, we have tried to keep the approach simple and accessible to the beginner. Before jumping into these special topics, we recommend that you acquaint yourself with the āsanas and prāṇāyāma presented in chapter 2, as well as the progression of learning, as we refer to them throughout this chapter. When following these guidelines, you might ask yourself: Which poses, or actions within a pose, give me the most insight into my condition? Do the recommended poses bring sensitivity to how I am feeling or adjusting the area of concern? Am I still able to work with my breath intelligently (as described in chapter 2)? As you become more confident, or if you have more experience, you may find many connections between the poses suggested here and more advanced āsanas or families of āsanas. As with all āsana, if anything causes pain, it is better to stop and seek the advice of a Certified Iyengar Yoga Teacher.

There are also several topics that we don't discuss here but that may be relevant for people experiencing pelvic floor pain. For example, irritable bowel syndrome (IBS), painful bladder syndrome (PBS) or interstitial cystitis (IC), endometriosis, polycystic ovarian syndrome (PCOS), and fibroids are all conditions that may cause secondary pelvic floor symptoms. Along with seeking medical treatment, we recommend following the guidelines given for Weeks 1 to 3 in chapter 2 of this book, as these sequences focus on softening the pelvic floor muscles, synchronizing the breath, and aligning the pelvis. Also see "Additional Resources" in the appendix, particularly *Geeta S. Iyengar's Guide to a Woman's Yoga Practice* by Lois Steinberg, which has helpful information about some of these conditions.

## Perineal Tears

As a baby passes through the vagina during childbirth, the tissue in the surrounding area needs to stretch enough to accommodate its shape and size. During this transition, tissue tearing may naturally occur at the labia minora, or more commonly at the perineal tissue, located between the anus and vaginal opening. Tears are common and can vary in their size and depth. They can be related to or determined by many factors, including the baby's position, a high birth weight, family history, the care provider, the setting, and whether the individual is having a first-time birthing experience. In some circumstances, forceps or a vacuum may be used to help deliver the baby, or an episiotomy, an intentional incision that extends the vaginal opening toward the anus, may be performed. In these cases, tearing may occur in deeper layers of tissue.

To prepare the tissue in this area for delivery, perineal massage can be performed within a few weeks prior to your due date. In addition, during labor and delivery, use of a warm compress over the perineum can help to prepare your tissue to lengthen and stretch. These practices can be useful in reducing the occurrence of a tear or the depth and degree of tearing when it does occur.

## Perineal Tears That Can Occur during Childbirth

Perineal tears related to childbirth are graded on a scale of 1 to 4, from superficial to deep. A 1st degree tear affects the perineal tissue. These tears are small and skin-deep. They often heal on their own in about six weeks without any method of closure required. Second degree tears also affect the perineal tissue, but they extend beyond the superficial skin and affect muscle tissue. These tears may require some intervention to help with closure, such as sutures, and typically heal within six to twelve weeks. On full closure of 1st and 2nd degree tears, external scar massage around and internal scar massage directly over the affected tissue is recommended, as discussed in detail next. Third degree tears are less common. They extend through the perineal area into the muscle around the anus and the external anal sphincter. Due to the length and depth of tissue affected, 3rd degree tears can affect bowel, bladder, and sexual activity, often leading to a reduction in muscle tension and strength. Sutures are required to promote healing, which often takes twelve weeks or more. Fourth degree tears extend beyond the musculature of the anus into the rectum and require more specialized surgical repair. This type of repair usually takes place in an operating room rather than a delivery room. Healing time for 4th degree

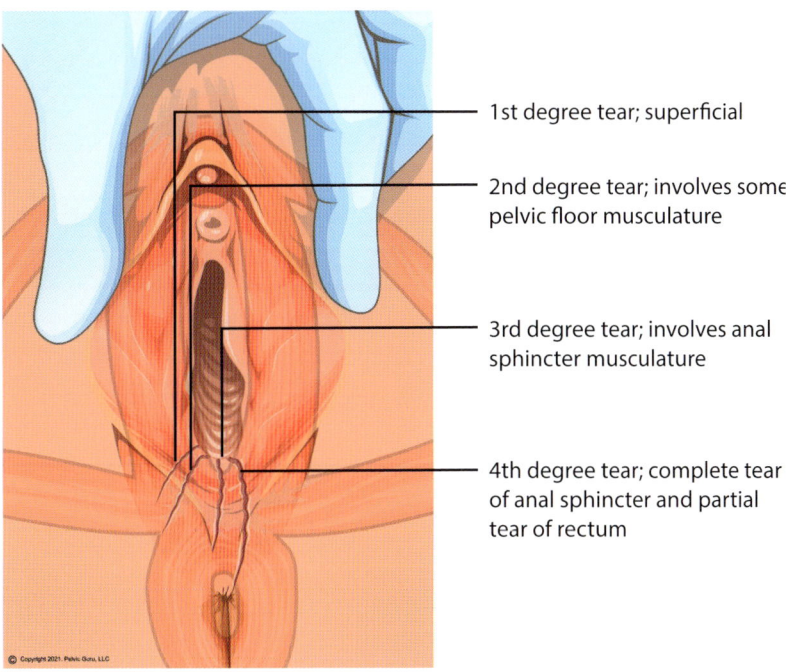

1st degree tear; superficial

2nd degree tear; involves some pelvic floor musculature

3rd degree tear; involves anal sphincter musculature

4th degree tear; complete tear of anal sphincter and partial tear of rectum

© Copyright 2021. Pelvic Guru, LLC

**FIGURE 3.1.**

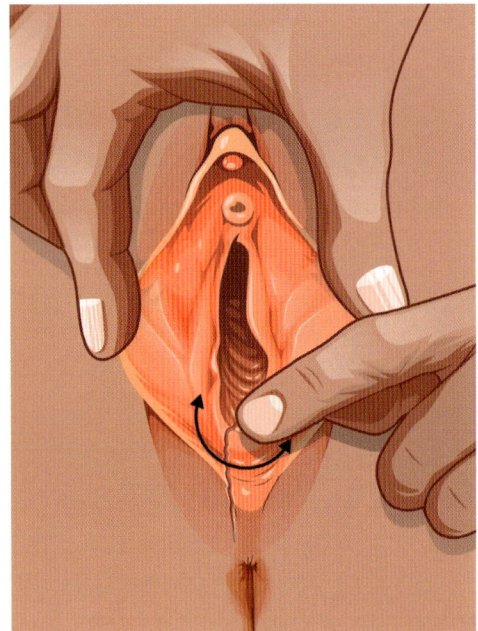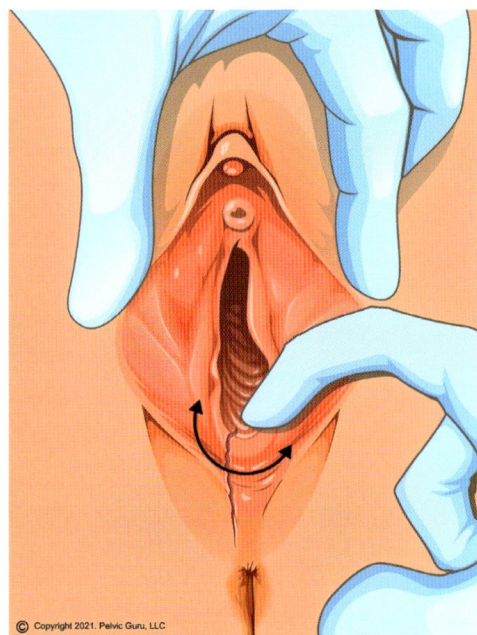

© Copyright 2021. Pelvic Guru, LLC

FIGURE 3.2. **Postpartum perineal scar massage.**

tears is individualized and generally takes months. Prior to doing any external or internal massage with 3rd and 4th degree repairs, obtain clearance from your qualified health care provider as they guide you through your recovery.

In the event of a tear, depending on the depth and degree of the tissue affected, the area will either be left open to heal on its own or will be closed with sutures. In either situation, scar tissue forms as a normal part of the body's natural healing process. During this process, the body produces a tough, fibrous material called collagen to fill in and eventually close the affected area. This tissue is weaker than the original tissue and will never reach the full strength of uninjured tissue. Since scar tissue has less elasticity than muscle, left unaddressed it can become stiff, contributing to limitations in movement and imbalance. This can lead to injury, pain, and difficulty with certain activities, including āsana practice, exercise, pleasurable touch, penetrative sex, or bowel movements. Scar massage is an effective tool to help mobilize this tissue so that it moves in a more efficient manner, similar to the movements of uninjured muscle tissue.

## Perineal Scar Massage

We've heard many students and clients say that no one told them they could do scar massage to help with healing or to reduce pain during postpartum recovery. Scar massage is appropriate at some point in the healing process for anyone who has sustained a tear during delivery. If scar massage is something you want to do on your own, it helps to have a sense of what you might be feeling. Generally, uninjured tissue tends to be soft and forgiving and will have a quality of rebound when you press and release it, whereas scar tissue usually does not. Scar tissue can be recognized as an area of dense, fibrous tissue that feels firm to touch compared with normal tissue. When you press on the tissue you might notice tenderness, pain, or even a slight burning feeling.

Once the tissue has healed and any open areas are closed, generally six to twelve weeks postpartum, you can begin scar massage directly over the affected area. Prior to that, you can gently touch and glide the skin just outside the affected area, but wait until it's closed completely for any direct contact with the scar itself. Scar massage can accelerate overall healing time and may provide great relief from related symptoms such as tension, aching, stiffness, or pain. Whether your scar is new or several years old, massaging your scar can help address present symptoms and can reduce the likelihood or severity of future issues.

## PERFORMING PERINEAL SCAR TISSUE MASSAGE

1. Wash your hands with soap and water.

2. Establish a quiet, comfortable environment without distraction (in bed, the shower, or the tub) and have coconut or vitamin E oil handy.

3. Sit with a pillow behind your back, with your knees bent, and move one knee out to the side, supporting it with a pillow.

4. Consider using a handheld mirror to look at the affected tissues and get a better idea of where to focus your massage.

5. Use some oil (avoid soap) on one or two fingertips and gently place them over or around the scar without any movement. Direct your breath toward your fingers, breathing into the area around the scar. If this is difficult or not tolerable, practice this for a few minutes daily until it becomes more comfortable.

6. Begin with light pressure. Slide your fingers back and forth in different directions: side to side, up and down, diagonally, clockwise, and counterclockwise.

7. Notice any specific areas of discomfort, heightened sensation, or stiffness. Spend a little more time massaging the tissue in these areas.

8. Gradually add more pressure as tolerated. You do not have to press so hard that you find yourself holding your breath, guarding, or clenching. Breathe steadily throughout the massage process and keep pain levels below a 3 out of 10.

9. If your scar extends into the vaginal opening or deep perineal tissue, you can insert one finger inside the vaginal opening and keep one finger over the perineum, imagining your fingers can touch. Slowly roll your fingers back and forth, gently lifting the tissue at the same time.

10. Continue this process for about five minutes, until the tissue feels less sensitive to touch and slightly easier to glide over and move.

11. Remove your fingers, and wash your hands with soap and water.

Notice whether you can detect any change with regard to movement or sensation in the areas you addressed. Changes may be noticeable right away, or they may require more time and repeated massage.

Repeat daily, every other day, or as often as you can based on your tolerance. Newly postpartum individuals may need more rest time between massages initially.

## Approach to Āsana

If tearing has occurred, it is extremely important that you approach your āsana practice slowly and sensitively. There is no āsana that will magically heal your tear, and you need to wait until the tear heals to do āsana. However, you may find that doing prāṇāyāma aids in the healing process. Start with Śavāsana on a bolster (see fig. 2.59), directing your breath to the affected area. Learn to synchronize your breath with the movements of the pelvic floor muscles as outlined in Weeks 1 to 3 in chapter 2, and focus your attention on inhaling while spreading and relaxing your pelvic floor. This attention to your breath can even be practiced in bed in the days immediately following birth, while you are resting and recovering. You may start to notice how the breath brings softness, blood flow, and elasticity back to the affected tissues. If the tear is particularly painful, you may notice muscles around the affected area gripping or tensing as a compensation or as a response to the pain. Using your breath to release gripping can be very soothing.

Once the tear itself and any sutures have healed, you can proceed with supported supine poses (see the Week 1 āsanas in chapter 2). Take care with any poses that spread the groin outward. For example, Supta Baddha Koṇāsana (fig. 2.2) is a beneficial pose during early postpartum recovery, but you may need bolsters or several pillows under your knees to lessen the stretch of the inner groins. In Supta Vīrāsana (fig. 2.7), a belt around the thighs can bring relief and relaxation to the inner groins and pelvic floor. As you continue your healing process, you may notice that there are imbalances between the two sides of the pelvis due to scar tissue and accompanying compensations. Take great care in any pose that spreads the legs apart laterally, especially standing poses that are weight-bearing. The scar tissue itself is weak and stiff, and the surrounding musculature may be tense. Notice whether you have more discomfort on one side, feelings of weakness or instability in the hip joint, or tension in the pelvic floor, buttocks, or lower back. These are signs that you may need to work with additional support: a wall, a trestle, or simply not going as deeply into the pose. Remember, you should still be able to breathe and connect with your pelvic floor as you move in and out of any āsana.

Tonifying both sides of the pelvic floor is very important to bring back stability and firmness to the whole pelvic area, including the hip, sacroiliac, and lumbar joints. Use the techniques provided in Weeks 3 and 4. Remember, scar tissue can be both weak and inflexible. Combining the tonifying actions in the poses given, along with the scar tissue massage described earlier, can have a powerful healing effect.

## Cesarean Birth

Birthing by cesarean section differs from a vaginal birth in many ways, mainly that a cesarean birth is a major surgery that directly affects the abdominal wall.

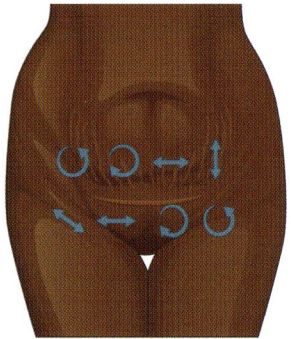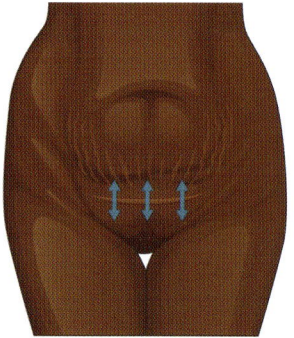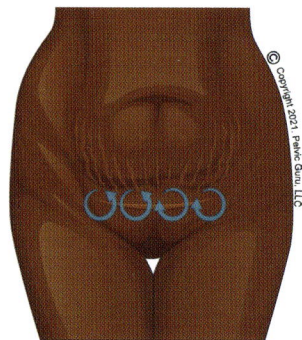

FIGURE 3.3. Cesarean section scar massage

Prior to birth, however, the effect of a full-term pregnancy on the pelvic floor muscles is the same, regardless of how someone gives birth. In other words, the pelvic floor muscles of a person who has a cesarean birth are also affected and deserve the same degree of attention and care as a person who births vaginally. Anyone who has experienced a cesarean birth can follow the general outline of care provided in chapter 2 and throughout this book, with some modifications. One thing that is different for a person who has had a cesarean birth is that the rate of healing is usually slower than with a vaginal birth. This is because more time is required to heal and begin recovery following this major abdominal surgical procedure. Initially, everyday movements like sitting up, rolling over, and carrying and lifting objects are limited based on possible post-surgical precautions, muscle weakness, and physical discomfort.

Similar to our earlier description of healing from perineal tearing, as tissue heals, scar tissue and adhesions can develop on or around the surrounding area, including tissues and organs of the pelvis: the uterus, ovaries, bladder, or colon. Over time, people may experience pulling sensations, stiffness, tension, or pain somewhere in the lower abdominal area. This can contribute to difficulty with everyday experiences (including wearing clothes comfortably), frequent urination, lower back pain, and exercise or doing movements that include lifting, squatting, or bending.

In the initial days and weeks following delivery, you can direct your breath toward your belly and offer light touch to your abdomen and tissue around the healing incision. This can help you reconnect physically with the site of tissue injury, assist with emotional healing, and bring the nervous system into a more balanced state. Once the external tissue is healed, usually around four to six weeks postpartum, you can begin scar massage to aid healing and support better movement and function.

## PERFORMING ABDOMINAL SCAR MASSAGE

1. Lie down in a comfortable and quiet environment with your legs supported by pillows or your knees bent, and your feet flat on the floor. Grab some coconut or vitamin E oil.

2. Consider looking at your scar and skin surrounding the area using a hand mirror to appreciate its size, shape, and appearance.

3. In the early stages, before the scar is healed completely on the outside, perform the following techniques above and below the scar but not directly over it.

4. Put some oil on your fingers and place your fingers somewhere on your scar. Move side to side, and up and down. Notice any areas that don't want to move or feel painful. It is OK if there is some discomfort, but avoid levels of pain that create clenching or guarding or cause you to hold your breath.

5. Once the deeper layers of the incision have completely healed, after about eight to ten weeks, you can apply more pressure and gradually sink farther into the tissue immediately beneath and surrounding your scar. Remain at a greater depth and continue to massage up and down, side to side, and add circles in clockwise and counterclockwise directions.

6. When you feel an area that is tense, pause here for a few seconds and wait until you feel a release or notice a change in the tissue tension.

7. As tissue becomes more malleable, you can begin to lift and roll it between your finger pads using your thumb on one side and your index and middle fingers on the other.

8. Once the tissue begins to move more freely, do the massage once a week. As the tissue begins to feel better and remains this way, repeat the massage once a month, or as needed.

For some people the incision and the area around it can be extra sensitive to touch. In this case you can practice reducing heightened sensitivity by rubbing around or directly on the affected area for five minutes a few times a day, using a cotton ball initially and progressively working up to coarser materials like a towel. Tapping the skin on or around the incision can also be useful. Work your way up to eventually massaging the tissue, gradually increasing the amount of pressure used.

## Approach to Āsana

While the approach to āsana following a cesarean birth is not radically different from that of a vaginal birth, there are some key differences, especially in the healing process. In general, healing from a cesarean takes longer. A cesarean is a major surgery, and like with any surgery, you may get easily fatigued. Simple things like walking or picking up and carrying a baby are tiring. While we've noted timing throughout chapter 2, in general, those recovering from a cesarean should wait until the incision is completely healed, about eight to ten weeks, before attempting any āsana. Supine prāṇāyāma, supported on a bolster or blankets (fig. 2.59), can be practiced sooner and may help you recover as you bring breath and fresh blood flow to the whole abdominal area. When you're ready to begin your practice of āsana, you may follow the steps laid out in chapter 2. You may feel that your pelvic floor does not need as much attention as someone who has experienced a vaginal birth, but, as described earlier, the pelvic floor is influenced by pregnancy itself, and learning to correctly relax and engage your pelvic floor muscles can influence intra-abdominal pressure.

Many people experience a greater degree of abdominal instability after a cesarean as compared to a vaginal birth. The recovery process will be slow and should not be rushed or forced. While we describe this process in great detail in chapter 2, especially in Weeks 5 and 6, you may find you need to wait even longer than suggested or go more slowly than you might initially assume. In general, you should focus on poses that create a gentle uḍḍīyāna bandha action; for example, you can start with supine poses and Mahā Mudrā (fig. 2.53), progressing to standing poses like Utkaṭāsana (fig. 2.88), and then proceeding with gentle abdominal poses like Ūrdhva Prasārita Pādāsana with the support of the wall (fig. 2.94), and Supta Pādāṇguṣṭhāsana I (fig. 2.96). It is important to learn the engagement of your transverse abdominis muscles, as described in Week 6, as this creates the foundation for additional stability. You may want to familiarize yourself with the section on the vāyus given in Week 5 as well as "Diaphragms, Breathing, and Pressures" in chapter 1. Also, read through "Diastasis Recti Abdominis" in this chapter, as some of the guidelines provided pertain to recovery from abdominal surgery.

# Pelvic Organ Prolapse

When defined by symptoms, pelvic organ prolapse (POP) has a prevalence of 3 to 6 percent and up to 50 percent when based on vaginal examination.[18] POP occurs when any of the pelvic organs—the vagina, bladder, urethra, uterus, rectum, and sometimes the small intestine—descend from their normal position by varying degrees (grades 0 to 4). When organs descend, they may bulge into another organ, and in some cases, as seen with grades 3 and 4, out of the vagina or anus.

As we noted in chapter 1, the pelvic organs are supported directly by the pelvic floor muscles, ligaments, and connective tissues. Wherever there are openings in the pelvic floor, for example, around the rectum and the vagina, there is less

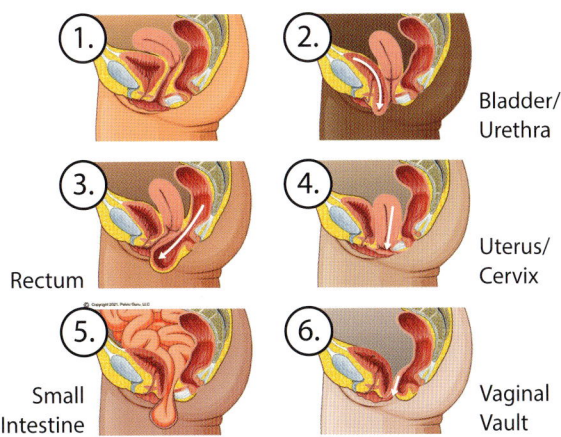

1.   Anatomy without prolapse
2.   Cystocele/cystourethrocele
3.   Rectocele
4.   Uterine prolapse
5.   Enterocele
6.   Vaginal vault prolapse

FIGURE 3.4.  **Variations in pelvic organ prolapse**

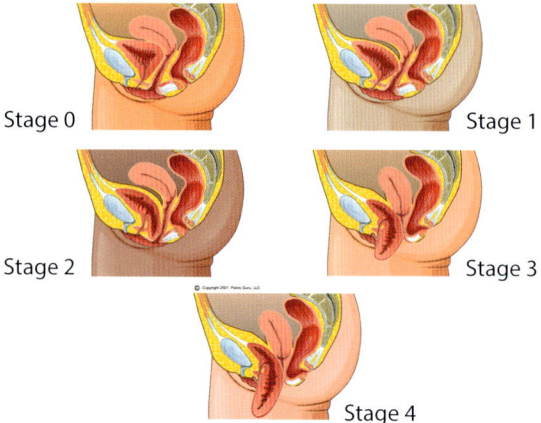

**FIGURE 3.5. Varying grades of bladder prolapse (cystocele)**

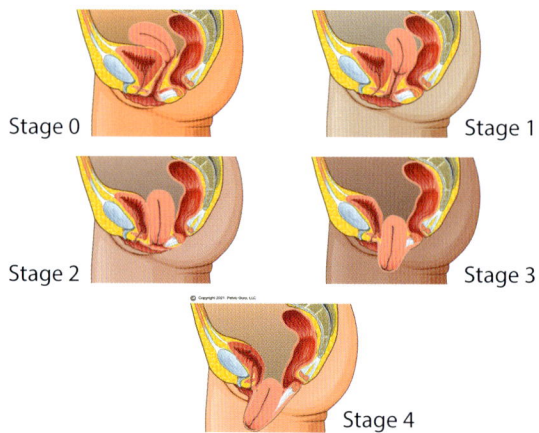

**FIGURE 3.6. Varying grades of uterine prolapse**

muscular support for the organs. In addition, pelvic muscle weakness, as well as tissue laxity resulting from elevated relaxin hormone levels, contribute to reduced organ support. Relaxin levels spike during the first trimester, and while they drop after delivery, overall relaxin remains elevated throughout the postpartum period until breastfeeding or chestfeeding ends. Organ prolapse can also be influenced by elevated abdominal and pelvic pressures that occur due to pregnancy, delivery, chronic constipation, frequent coughing, posture and alignment changes, hysterectomy, and hormonal changes associated with menopause.

Recognizable signs and symptoms from your body could tip you off as to whether you have a prolapse. Some of these include urinary or fecal leaking, incomplete bladder or bowel emptying, or the need to splint in order to empty.

Splinting refers to the use of your finger or fingers either externally at the perineal body or internally through the vaginal canal to support or move organs or surrounding tissues to allow for more complete bladder or bowel emptying. Other symptoms associated with prolapse can include back pain and discomfort with penetration or intercourse. Some people with prolapse describe a generally looser feeling inside and vaginal flatulence (air that makes a sound as it exits the vagina) with some forms of exercise and activity. Additionally, you might feel heaviness or pressure in the pelvic floor.

There are some simple nonsurgical steps you can take to begin addressing prolapse. These include making sure you have plenty of fiber and water in your diet to reduce constipation, and adapting exercise and weight lifting of any kind to avoid straining. Additionally, it can be beneficial to learn how to breathe effectively to reduce and manage pressures that act on the abdomen and pelvis. You should determine whether pelvic floor strengthening is right for you and how to do it effectively as described throughout this book. Breathing and working with pelvic floor contractions can be done with the pelvis in an elevated position so that gravity aids in the process (fig. 3.7). The use of a pessary, a support device that can be inserted through the vagina to help support the pelvic floor organs, can help to manage and even reduce prolapse over time.

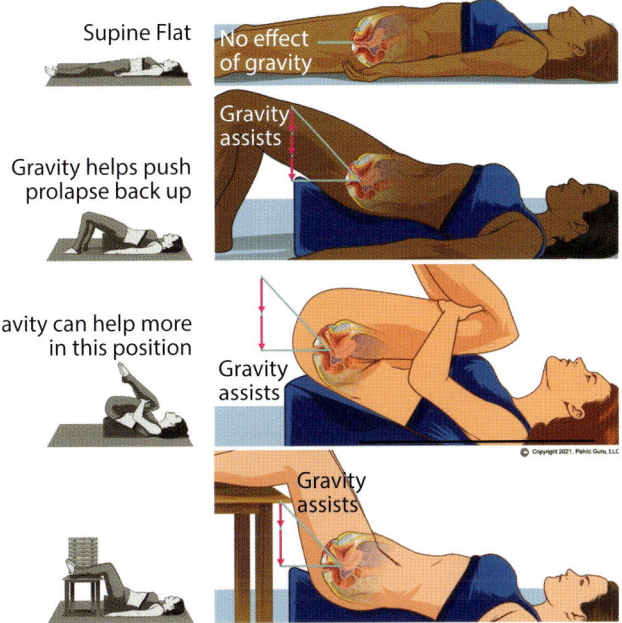

**FIGURE 3.7.** Positions for healing pelvic organ prolapse

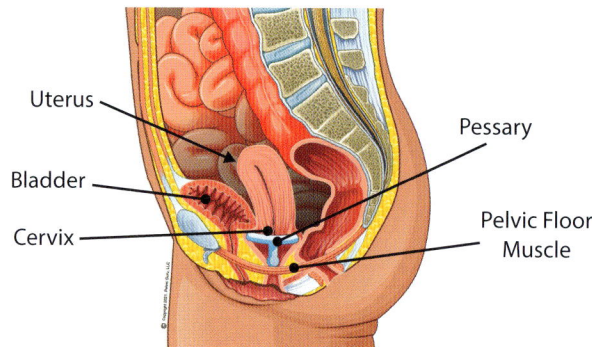

FIGURE 3.8. **Pessary for pelvic organ prolapse**

During movement and exercise such as yoga, consideration should be taken throughout pregnancy and the postpartum period to avoid overstretching or straining already compromised tissues. Gaining a better understanding of factors that contribute to and affect your prolapse through education and training with a qualified health care provider or movement specialist is essential for effective long-term management.

## Approach to Āsana

When working with yoga students, organ prolapse is one of the most common complaints we hear about. Some may be new parents experiencing it for the first time after pregnancy and delivery and feel alarmed about it, while some have been living with prolapse for some time and feel resigned to it. While prolapse is common, the good news is that there are many yoga tools you can use to reduce or fully remedy your prolapse.

Organ prolapse can be caused and aggravated by excessive downward pressure on the organs. We can think of this as an excess of, or disruption to, apāna vāyu, the downward-moving energy that controls elimination and childbirth, among other things (see Week 5). Those who experience prolapse know that anything that exerts downward force, like coughing, sneezing, jumping, or running, can exacerbate symptoms. Breathing patterns and diaphragm movements that are not coordinated with pelvic floor movements, that create more pressure by overinflating the abdomen and pushing the breath downward, or that are restricted to the abdomen without breathing into the chest can also be a hindrance to relieving the pressure on the organs.

As advised in our Week 1 sequence, if you are newly postpartum you may have several weeks of bleeding and discharge. During this time that you are still healing, it can be frustrating only to focus on very gentle supported postures and breathing. However, you may find relief by doing Supta Baddha Koṇāsana using the cone (fig. 2.43), as this brings the pelvis into alignment, moves the tailbone inward, and helps the organs move back and inward toward the sacrum. The sacrum acts as a bed for the organs, helping them come back to their correct position.

Once your bleeding has completely stopped, the inverted poses, practiced safely and with support, can provide immediate and powerful relief to those experiencing prolapse as they literally invert the pelvis, changing the relationship of the pelvis and organs to gravity. You may actually feel your organs shift back into position, or you may feel relief from the associated heaviness and pressure. Starting with Viparīta Karaṇī with either bent or straight legs (figs. 2.23 and 2.175) and Sālamba Sarvāṅgāsana using the wall (fig. 2.34), build up your timing in these āsanas. A helpful version of Nirālamba Sarvāṅgāsana and Koṇāsana in Sarvāṅgāsana is given in Week 7 (figs. 2.173 and 2.174), although it requires some familiarity and comfort with the props. If you practiced Śīrṣāsana (fig. 2.102) prior to pregnancy, you can begin to incorporate it back into your practice, but you may need to wait some weeks before you feel strong enough to kick up. Once all three poses are familiar and comfortable, reverse the order in your daily practice: Śīrṣāsana, Sālamba Sarvāṅgāsana, then Viparīta Karaṇī.

The other important tool that yoga offers us is the coordinated effort of mūla bandha and uḍḍīyāna bandha. In the Week 2 sequence, work with the brick between your legs in Tāḍāsana to learn how to engage the legs in lifting the pelvis and the pelvic organs up. Then proceed with the other standing poses in Week 2, being mindful that no downward pressure is being created. While these poses don't teach mūla bandha and uḍḍīyāna bandha specifically, they pave the way for later learning. Week 3 begins our practice of mūla bandha, and although it's helpful, you should start slowly and not do too much in one sitting. Further, sitting too long may exacerbate symptoms. Start by practicing mūla bandha in reclined or supine positions. Then try gently practicing mūla bandha during your standing poses and in your inversions. Try just a few repetitions of mūla bandha, holding for only a few moments. This is challenging, but you may find you make progress quickly! With patience and perseverance, you will slowly build awareness and endurance.

Uḍḍīyāna bandha is introduced in Week 5. Start with Ūrdhva Prasārita Pādāsana with the legs at 90 degrees supported by the wall (fig. 2.94) and Adho Mukha Śvānāsana with the feet on blocks or a stool (fig. 2.86) or with the full setup using ropes, a Siṁhāsana box, and blocks (fig. 2.154). While Ūrdhva Prasārita Pādāsana requires more intentional abdominal lifting, and may be challenging if there is a lot of weakness in the core, Adho Mukha Śvānāsana, especially the version supported with ropes and height under the feet, creates a natural suctioning feeling of uḍḍīyāna bandha with very little effort. Both should be utilized to bring understanding to the synchronized effort of the breath, the abdominal walls, and the organs.

Another useful tool is learning how to engage your transverse abdominis muscles. The transverse abdominis muscle is the deepest layer of the abdominal or core muscles and helps stabilize the abdomen, lumbar spine, and pelvis (see chapter 1). Start by following the description of how to engage the transverse abdominis in Week 6 in Ardha Setubandha (fig. 2.111), as well as in Ūrdhva Prasārita Pādāsana (fig. 2.94). Many people are eager to do sit-ups or similar strengthening exercises to tone their core; the problem is that it can easily create excessive downward pressure onto the pelvic organs, further exacerbating symptoms. The combined actions of engaging the transverse abdominis along with the bandhas gives an upward lift to the pelvic organs and elongates and broadens the abdominal muscles even while engaging (eccentric contraction). This requires a lot of concentration!

Those who are newly postpartum may be surprised how challenging this coordinated effort feels, but with even a few weeks of practice, you may notice more stability and control coming in the poses as well as in your daily activities. Until the prolapse has improved, you need to be cautious about doing any other deeper abdominal āsanas, deep backbends, or any pose where downward pressure is felt. Once you feel more stable in your deeper core muscles and your prolapse has improved, you can continue with the other abdominal āsanas presented in Weeks 5 and 6, but you may need to go very slowly, working in stages, so that the stabilizing actions described above are not lost.

## Diastasis Recti Abdominis

Diastasis recti abdominis (DRA) is a separation of the linea alba, a thickened fascial band formed by the connective tissue of the three underlying layers of abdominal muscle (transverse abdominis, internal oblique, and external oblique). The linea alba runs vertically down the midline of the abdomen from the xiphoid process at the bottom of the sternum to the pubic symphysis at the top of the pelvis, connecting the left and right sides of the most superficial layer of abdominal muscle, the rectus abdominis (see fig. 1.23). It is through this connection that the two sides of the abdomen can communicate during movement so they can coordinate their actions.

While DRA is a common condition that many people develop during pregnancy or within a few weeks postpartum, it is important to note that regardless of gender or age, some gapping is actually normal. Without a little space available for your tissues to move, imagine what would happen at your abdomen every time it expands and relaxes when you breathe. Or consider how you would feel after eating a large meal if there were no relief mechanism built in (unbuttoning your pants will only get you so far)! There needs to be some give and the linea alba allows for this.[19]

During pregnancy, as a result of pressure on the abdominal wall and the abdominal muscles adapting to the shape and size of a growing fetus, this separation can expand enough to delay, interrupt, or cut off communication and coordination between the right and left sides of your abdomen. Additional factors that contribute to the development of a DRA include hormonal elastic changes on the linea alba, the weight of the baby, cesarean birth, two or more pregnancies, being age thirty-five or older at the time of delivery, and carrying multiple babies.[20] While most of these factors aren't under your control, there are things that you can be aware of and that can influence DRA. These include your exercise and movement habits during pregnancy, your posture, avoiding activities or exercises that cause straining or bulging of your abdominal muscles, and excessive weight gain.

DRA can occur in different places along the linea alba, including at the navel, above or below the navel, or throughout the full length of the linea alba (fig. 3.9).

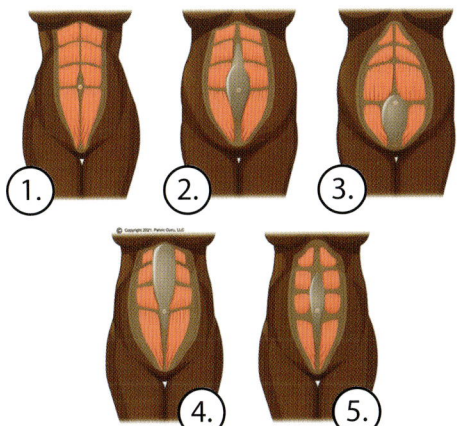

1. Abdomen without diastasis

2. Diastasis around umbilicus

3. Below umbilicus diastasis

4. Above umbilicus diastasis

5. Diastasis along full length of linea alba

**FIGURE 3.9. Variations of diastasis recti abdominis**

Some signs that point to a separation include seeing or feeling a gap along your midline, a visible bulge or "pooch" just above or below your navel, or the appearance of coning or doming when you contract your abdominal muscles. If you have a DRA, you may feel weak and "jelly-like" at your core, and DRA can also be accompanied by other symptoms, like urinary incontinence; lower back, pelvis, or hip pain; or hernias.

When determining whether you have a separation and how to approach healing, it is most important to restore tension to the fascia, as this will permit communication and coordination throughout your movement systems. This factor is more important than whether or not a separation closes completely. While some degree of closure is important and can affect the appearance of your abdomen, research has shown a variation in normal width measurements from 0 to 35 millimeters along the linea alba in women who have never had children. Therefore, the presence of some amount of gap is considered normal.[21]

Each person has an individualized set of factors that influences their DRA recovery, including hormonal changes related to breastfeeding or chestfeeding, or genetic factors that influence tissue integrity. In some cases, connection may be restored and reintegrated with the rest of the core on its own or within a short amount of time. For others, it takes months or longer to adequately restore this connection. If tension of the connective tissue inside the gap is poor and unable to be restored with targeted exercises and rehabilitation, it is possible that symptoms will not resolve, and other ways of creating tension may be considered, such as surgery.

Next we've given some guidelines on how to screen yourself for a DRA. When intact, the linea alba should feel somewhat firm and tensioned, like a trampoline. If you have a diastasis, the tissue may feel thinned out, a bit like cellophane. After screening yourself, if your fingers can sink into your abdominal cavity past the abdominal muscles, or if you can fit two and a half or more fingers width between the borders of your rectus abdominis, you may want to adjust your practice in order to address the separation. You may also want to seek additional guidance from a qualified health care or movement professional or pelvic physical therapist.

If you suspect or have already confirmed that you have a DRA, there are movement patterns and habits to modify or be aware of so that you can remain active without making things worse. To begin with, practice steady breathing. This applies to toileting habits and movement alike. Avoid holding your breath, since it creates an increase in intra-abdominal pressure. Instead, practice using an exhalation whenever you exert effort, change positions, or lift anything.

Approach twists with an understanding of the different movements that occur at your thoracic spine (rotation) and lumbar spine (flexion and extension). Twisting through your thoracic spine is necessary to maintain spinal health, while twisting into your lumbar spine can slow DRA healing and lead to future movement problems. Learn how to move your thoracic spine separately from your lumbar. Avoid positions and movements that place additional strain on your abdomen and its fasciae. Examples of more demanding movements are push-ups and sit-ups and other strong abdominal movements. If you have a DRA, you must first learn how to generate enough fascial tension to reconnect the two sides of your body to allow for effective and efficient transmission of forces. Usually, movements that place mild to moderate demand on your fascial system are a good place to begin before asking and expecting your body to work well in more demanding positions.[22]

## HOW TO SCREEN YOURSELF FOR A DRA

1. Lie on your side and roll onto your back with your knees bent.
2. Place the pads of two or three fingers directly on your skin over your navel, with your fingerpads facing toward your pelvis.
3. Press down and raise your head and the top of your shoulder blades off the floor as if doing a mini sit-up.
   - What happens at the moment you raise your head?
   - Do you notice muscles begin to grip your fingers?
   - How many fingers can you fit into the gap between the muscles, and how deep can you press?
   - Do you notice any tenting, doming, or coning of your abdomen?
4. Lower your head and shoulders, move your hand three finger widths above your navel, and test again.
5. Lower your head and shoulders, move your hand three finger widths below your navel, and test again.

## Approach to Āsana

When adjusting your practice to address a diastasis, it is important to stay focused on the deeper goal. Many students want a cosmetic fix. However, the goal should be to create stability in the deeper layers of the abdominal wall and provide support for the spine and the organs. Many students want to start strengthening their abdominals right away by doing sit-ups or similar exercises. However, these exercises only affect the most superficial layers of the abdominal wall, and because the diastasis is occurring in these layers, doing this kind of superficial strengthening can actually put excessive pressure on the diastasis and make it worse. Instead, focus on engaging the transverse abdominis muscles, the deepest layer of the abdominal wall, and coordinating them with steady breathing to establish a stable foundation.

After confirming that you have a diastasis by using the screening instructions provided earlier or by seeing your provider, begin with the breath instructions given in the Week 1 sequence. Pay particular attention to the inhalation, making sure that as you spread your diaphragm and lower ribs, you are not pushing the breath down into the abdomen. As you breathe out, notice how the exhalation naturally brings the two sides of the abdominal wall toward each other. Once a natural rhythm can be felt, try extending the exhalation (Ujjāyī II) to emphasize this movement. This way of breathing can be attempted in any of the Week 1 poses. Gentle stretching is fine, but if supine poses such as Supta Baddha Koṇāsana on a bolster (fig. 2.2) feel too intense, try moving the bolster slightly up toward your head side so that your thoracic spine can lengthen away from the lumbar spine and your abdomen does not get pushed. You may also find more relief in the supine poses by using a transverse bolster under your thoracic spine with plenty of head support, as this gives more lift of the chest away from the abdomen.

Once you've established your breath, you can proceed with the sequences of āsanas as they are presented in chapter 2. To help aid your recovery, you may want to familiarize yourself with the section on bandhas in Week 3, in particular, the action of lifting the abdomen as in uḍḍīyāna bandha, presented in the instructions for pose 2, Mahā Mudrā (fig. 2.53). This work can be deepened in poses like Tāḍāsana (fig. 2.60), Vṛkṣāsana (fig. 2.67), Utthita Trikoṇāsana (fig. 2.68), Utkaṭāsana (fig. 2.88), and the first stage of Ūrdhva Prasārita Pādāsana with support (fig. 2.94), given in Weeks 4 and 5. Also familiarize yourself with the section on the vāyus given in Week 5 as well as "Diaphragms, Breathing, and Pressures" in chapter 1. These sections describe in various ways how to reduce downward pressure in the abdomen that can exacerbate your diastasis. Once you can begin to feel how your breath is moving in the various āsanas, you will start to notice the effect it has on the vāyus and on your intra-abdominal pressure. This will give you the sensitivity you need to move on in your āsana practice and your daily activities. At first it may seem like a lot of attention and effort is needed, but eventually these movements will become natural and effortless.

It's important not to jump to doing abdominal work right away, as the work done in sitting, standing, and inverted postures will all start to work on the stability of the core. However, you may want to review the instructions given in Week 6, pose 1, Ardha Setubandha, for how to engage the transverse abdominis muscles. Start by simply lying flat with bent knees and, feeling with your fingertips, engage the transverse abdominis muscles. This may take some practice, and you may feel that one side engages better than the other. Once you can feel these muscles, shift the pelvis posteriorly, trying to utilize the TA muscles in this action. Once you feel confident in this movement, you can also start to engage the buttocks and hamstrings, which will deepen the movement; however, they should not take over the work of the TA muscles.

You may want to stay with these small movements for several weeks before attempting additional abdominal postures. Slowly, over time, you can start to add in the other abdominal postures given in Week 6, such as the stages of Ūrdhva Prasārita Pādāsana (poses 2 to 4), staying with the supported versions of the āsanas for some time. Another pose that is particularly helpful is Nāvāsana with the support of the wall and a chair (fig. 2.136). Some students are surprised at how long it takes to gain strength and stability in the abdominal core, but patience and repetition are key here, rather than strong forceful effort. With time you will begin to feel more stable and confident not just in your āsanas but in your daily movements as well.

## Hernia

Following pregnancy and birth, you may notice a bump in your abdomen caused by a hernia. A hernia may develop due to increased pressures on the abdominal wall over the course of pregnancy, or during vaginal or cesarean births. These pressures can stretch and weaken abdominal muscles, or even cause tissues to thin in some areas. When this happens, inner intestinal lining, fat, or intestines can push up against these weakened areas and create a bump or a hernia. Postpartum hernias may develop around the navel because this part of the abdomen is naturally weaker than the rest of the abdominal wall. Similarly, a hernia may develop around the incision on a person who has had a cesarean birth as initially this tissue is weaker or may be subjected to elevated pressures from certain movements or activities prior to the tissue and muscles being fully healed.

If a hernia is small and does not cause pain, it's likely that no surgical intervention is needed. Similar to our discussion of both pelvic organ prolapse and diastasis recti abdominis, you will want to learn how to move, bend, lift, exercise, and breathe safely and efficiently, in ways that avoid excessive abdominal or pelvic pressure. Allow time for your body to heal following pregnancy and birth and avoid intense exercise, heavy lifting, or any activities that put pressure on your abdomen and pelvis. If you're experiencing constipation, take care not to push or hold your breath, which can create too much downward pressure. In addition to the āsana guidelines here, a physical therapist can guide you in doing gentle core exercises that will stabilize the abdominal area.

## Approach to Āsana

Similar to your approach to working with pelvic organ prolapse and diastasis recti abdominis, it may be helpful to think about the approach to working with a hernia in terms of pressures that may be present at the site of the hernia, as well as the stability and integrity of the underlying musculature. You should read through both the earlier sections as we focus on how to coordinate the movements of the breath to improve the relationship between intra-abdominal and pelvic pressures. Practices such as uḍḍīyāna bandha can bring tremendous relief of symptoms. For postpartum people in particular, a hernia can result from weakened or stretched abdominal tissue. Therefore, you need to work intelligently and sensitively to stabilize the deeper abdominal muscles.

Standing, seated, and inverted āsanas are all beneficial and will build up the strength in the legs and spine to maintain the lift of the chest, essential in remedying unnecessary pressure on the abdomen. Mahā Mudrā (fig. 2.53), Ūrdhva Prasārita Pādāsana 90 degrees with the legs supported at the wall (fig. 2.94), Nāvāsana at the wall with the support of a chair (fig. 2.136), and Ardha Setubandha (fig. 2.111) will all build the strength and stability needed to slowly reknit the muscle fibers together, creating abdominal wall support. Unsupported backward extensions should be avoided until the hernia has resolved as it is very difficult to control the abdominal pressure in these āsanas and students with a hernia may actually notice that the hernia bulges or "pops out" as soon as they go into a backbend. Once some stability is regained, supported Dwipāda Viparīta Daṇḍāsana (fig. 2.164) may be an appropriate backward extension to begin with, as the abdominal area is relatively neutral and the support of the chair will allow you to observe your breath and abdomen. This pose gives you the time and support needed to learn to move your abdomen back and up, relaxing any unnecessary pushing. This supported backward extension also teaches the opening of the thoracic spine, which is helpful in relieving overworking in the lumbar spine. Freedom in the chest will also bring freedom in the diaphragm, thus benefiting the overall coordination of breath, posture, and pressures.

# Urinary Issues

Urinary incontinence refers to an uncontrolled loss of urine. It is one of the most common reasons people seek out help for their pelvic floor. There are many different types of urinary incontinence and voiding dysfunctions, including stress urinary incontinence (SUI), urgency and frequency, mixed incontinence, overactive bladder (OAB), urinary hesitancy, and incomplete emptying. Understanding your specific symptoms is important because approaches to treatment may vary.

Stress urinary incontinence occurs when urine leaks out of the bladder involuntarily, usually with sudden physical movement or activity. The volume of urine lost can range from a small dribble to a much larger amount. This can be a result of elevated amounts of pressure from the abdomen on the bladder and urethra, causing the urethral sphincter, the muscle around the urethra, to briefly open. This may occur due to changes in the position of the organs or pelvic muscle weakness or tension. Other causes of pelvic floor muscle dysfunction that contribute to SUI are perineal injury or tears during childbirth, injury or trauma such as pelvic fracture, surgery in the vagina or rectum, and lack of exercise combined with increased time spent sitting.[23] Common events or activities that result in sudden, elevated abdominal and bladder pressures are coughing, laughing, jumping, running, heavy lifting, and sneezing.

Treatment for SUI may ultimately include Kegel exercises aimed at improving strength and coordination of the pelvic floor muscles (see Week 3 in chapter 2); however, as is the case with all muscles in the body, adequate muscle length must be available prior to beginning strengthening, as we describe throughout this book. A shortened or tightened muscle cannot contract effectively if it is unable to lengthen completely. In other words, it is an oversimplification to say that incontinence is due to weak pelvic floor muscles. Identifying and learning to release tension is an important first step in reeducating the pelvic floor muscles. Once these muscles are able to lengthen and move through their full range of motion, you can then begin strengthening. It is important to begin in positions with adequate support, and gradually transition to more challenging positions, and from static to dynamic movements. For some people, the use of graded pelvic weights that are inserted into the vagina can be useful for training the pelvic floor muscles (see "Additional Resources" in the appendix).

Urinary frequency occurs when voiding happens more frequently than deemed normal by the individual during waking hours.[24] While there are variations in what constitutes "normal," generally a person should be able to retain urine for two to four hours. Often, frequency is accompanied by urinary urgency, a strong need to urinate that can be painful or difficult to stop. This sensation can result in frequent trips to the bathroom or leakage before making it to the bathroom. When urgency and frequency are experienced together, it is called mixed incontinence. Urinary frequency may also be a sign of infection, such as a urinary tract infection (UTI), or can be related to sensitivity or quantities of certain foods and drinks.

Unintentional loss of urine may be caused by involuntary contraction of the bladder muscle, called the detrusor, and can result in an overactive bladder (OAB). A person with an overactive bladder feels the need to empty often throughout the day and may wake to empty more than once at night. This can be experienced whether or not the bladder is full. With both urinary urgency and an overactive bladder, anxiety may increase the urge to empty the bladder. The pelvic floor muscles may also become gripped over time as a defense against the feeling that you may leak urine, or as a response to pain in the bladder. This may then in turn contribute to increased symptoms of urgency, setting up an uncoordinated feedback loop within the nervous system.

There are a few approaches that you might take to address urinary frequency and urgency. Determining the cause of weakness or lack of coordination is necessary to determine the best course of treatment. As described above, you must first determine whether there is too much tension in the pelvic floor, and if so, addressing that tension is paramount. Eventually, a strong, coordinated contraction of the pelvic floor muscles can decrease the urge to urinate as well as help to keep the urethra closed.

Another important approach is to reeducate the bladder, especially if urgency and frequency are chronic. If you seek out a bathroom immediately when you notice the first urge, or as a "just in case" habit before you even get an urge, your bladder will become sensitive to small amounts of urine in the bladder and send unreliable signals that send you looking for a bathroom before your bladder is even halfway full. Normally an urge will be signaled when the bladder is 50 percent full. Allowing this initial urge to pass will allow the bladder to continue filling. When the next urge is signaled, the bladder will be about 75 percent full and the urge may be more persistent; this is a good time to seek out a bathroom. Over time, urgency will decrease as your bladder becomes accustomed to filling more completely before voiding.

Other types of urinary symptoms are urinary hesitancy, when one has difficulty initiating the flow of urine, and urinary intermittency, when the urinary stream is interrupted. Since the pelvic floor and bladder have a reciprocal relationship, when you sit down to urinate, the bladder, which is controlled by the detrusor muscle, contracts to empty the urine. The pelvic floor muscles should be relaxed to allow this to happen. When the relationship between the pelvic floor muscles and bladder is no longer coordinated due to elevated pelvic floor muscle tension, spasm, or behavioral habits, the pelvic floor muscles will inhibit the bladder contraction by not fully relaxing, causing difficulty or hesitancy in starting the urine stream. Using your breath to relax the pelvic floor muscles on the inhalation can help the bladder fully empty. Also, when seated on a toilet, bending forward with your legs spread wide apart, elbows resting on your knees, will lengthen and spread the pelvic floor muscles, allowing the bladder to empty urine more easily and completely. Avoid pushing or bearing down to empty the bladder, as this will increase downward pressure and can contribute to inefficient emptying.

## Approach to Āsana

The approach in yoga to incontinence and bladder issues in general can be tricky because several factors need to be taken into consideration to determine the best course of action. Some of these factors might include pelvic tension (see chapter 1), organ position, amount of time postpartum, age, whether you are pre- or postmenopausal, and your behavioral patterns. In general, it may help you to first determine your own pelvic floor landscape, as we've described throughout this book. Do you have elevated or low tension in the pelvic floor muscles? If there is an obvious answer to this question, that may be your first clue in resolving the incontinence.

As described earlier, elevated or high tension may be creating tension on the bladder itself. You may have difficulty voiding completely due to the inability to fully relax. A heightened sensitivity due to areas of high tone may give the feeling that you have to pee even if you've just gone to the bathroom. In these cases, start with the āsanas and breathing exercises presented in Week 1, focusing your attention on relaxation with the inhalation. Breathing can be especially helpful to practice while sitting on the toilet to ensure that the bladder and pelvic floor muscles are relaxing completely.

Alternatively, decreased tension may be at play, especially with stress incontinence. If you have low tension in the pelvic floor muscles, you should focus on mūla bandha and uḍḍīyāna bandha, inversions, the alignment of legs and pelvis in standing poses, and supine poses (see the cone adjustment in Week 2, pose 8). Start with the poses that are easiest for you and require the least amount of effort so that you can focus on your breathing and on the correct engagement of the pelvic floor muscles. Also pay attention to *where* you are contracting. In reviewing the anatomy of the pelvic floor muscles in chapter 1, it may be helpful to visualize the pelvic floor as a diamond shape composed of a front and back triangle. For some individuals, contraction of the muscles may be occurring predominantly in one triangle and not the other. For example, if the urethral sphincter is weak and you try to contract the pelvic floor, you may end up contracting the anal sphincter (posterior triangle of the pelvic floor) more than the urethral sphincter (anterior triangle of the pelvic floor). Try relaxing the anus and focus your efforts on the front triangle instead (see the section on aśvini mudrā and vajrolī mudrā, "Pelvic Floor Contractions and Bandhas," in Week 3). Once you feel some progress, gradually increase the intensity of the poses, while maintaining the contraction of the pelvic floor. It is not necessary to hold the contraction the entire duration of the pose, but you should work your way up to holding the contraction steadily for three or four seconds, then releasing completely before trying again. Intensity of the pose specifically refers to how much *downward pressure* is created by the pose. For example, jumping your legs apart for standing poses may be one of the most challenging actions for stress incontinence and may take many months or longer to accomplish without leaking. Again, you shouldn't rush to do more intense actions but should focus on the steady and even engagement and lift of the pelvic floor muscles through a variety of different movements.

# Vaginal Flatulence

We think it's fair to say that few things are as surprising as when air makes an unplanned exit through the vaginal canal, as in the case of vaginal flatulence (colloquially called "queefing" by some). While this phenomenon is certainly not limited to the postpartum population, it is commonly reported and experienced following pregnancy and birth. Common as it may be, it can become frustrating or feel embarrassing when it happens.

Following vaginal birth, the vaginal canal and pelvic muscles that surround the levator hiatus may be overstretched. When pelvic muscle strength and coordination are compromised and the vaginal canal is vacuous, it can be difficult to detect and prevent air from entering. During dynamic movement such as kicking up into Adho Mukha Vṛkṣāsana (Handstand), lifting a heavy weight, intercourse, or when simply moving from a seated to a standing position, air may be able to escape without warning. Some conditions, such as pelvic organ prolapse or procedures like a hysterectomy that result in a change in position and support of the pelvic organs, can also contribute to the occurrence of vaginal flatulence.

It is not only people with pelvic tissue and muscle stretching who experience vaginal flatulence. Those with tight pelvic floor muscles may also be affected since the muscles are unable to fully relax or contract effectively. Tight pelvic floor muscles can create a suctioning effect that brings air into the vagina, and when the trapped air is released, it often makes a sound. If you have had a cesarean birth, intra-abdominal pressure changes and pelvic muscle dysfunction can also be contributing factors. Additionally, hormonal fluctuations can play a role in vaginal flatulence. During the phases of ovulation and menstruation, while breastfeeding or chestfeeding, or during or after menopause, hormonal changes occur that contribute to connective tissue laxity.

For some people, vaginal flatulence resolves on its own within a few months of delivery. For others, pelvic floor therapy and eventually strengthening these muscles can be an effective way to reduce and manage this occurrence. Additionally, coordinating your exhale with your pelvic floor and deep abdominal muscles, the transverse abdominals, as described throughout this book, can be a useful strategy to practice integrating into your movements.

## Approach to Āsana

While vaginal flatulence can be embarrassing for some practitioners, let us reiterate that it is a common occurrence and does not necessarily indicate any deeper problem. Especially for those who have given birth vaginally multiple times, the space of the vaginal vault, the deep end of the vaginal canal, may be wider and the tissue less elastic than prior to birthing babies. You may also notice that the tendency toward flatulence changes with your menstrual cycle, becoming more pronounced just before, during, or just after your period. Vaginal flatulence may also be related in part to low tension in the pelvic floor muscles, and strengthening the pelvic floor muscles as we've described throughout this book may be an appropriate course of action.

Students most often experience vaginal flatulence when they are inverted, kicking up with one leg, taking the legs apart during an inversion, or when lowering one leg in an inversion. In short, during these actions, the opening to the vaginal canal is being stretched. Depending on the size of this opening and the degree to which one is stretching, the opening becomes wide enough to draw air into the vagina. Sometimes that air gets pushed out quickly with force, as when kicking up into an inversion. Sometimes the air coming in isn't as noticeable and only comes out noisily when the student comes down from the inversion. In either case, it can be a loud and embarrassing moment! One approach is to slow down any movement, usually in the legs, so that you can control your pelvic floor muscles. For example, in Śīrṣāsana, place your feet on a chair and slowly raise one leg at a time from the chair so that both the stretch and force is lessened. Additionally, mūla bandha can be beneficial here. Exhale and engage mūla bandha while you stretch one leg up if you are coming up into the inversion or while taking one leg down if you are coming out of the inversion. This is challenging to do with the legs apart! Over time and with practice, you may feel that you can better control the passing of air while taking your legs through a variety of movements.

## Painful Intercourse

Deciding when to return to having intercourse after birthing a baby is an individual and personal decision each person should make for themselves. While it is common to have a follow-up with your provider around six weeks after you give birth, this timeline is arbitrary and does not necessarily mean that all systems are go! Additional time for healing may be indicated on a physical, energetic, emotional, or mental level. Only you can decide when that time is. Some people return to pleasurable intercourse early in their recovery without too many challenges, but many others report feeling discomfort or experience pain with their initial attempts, especially during interceptive or penetrative intercourse. We often work with individuals who are not postpartum but are experiencing painful intercourse, often along with other pelvic floor symptoms. The American College of Obstetricians and Gynecologists reports that three out of four women experience painful sex at some point in their lives.[25] While painful intercourse is common, whether you are postpartum or not, keep in mind that pain with intercourse is never normal and should always be addressed.

Factors that may contribute to pain during intercourse include vaginal dryness or tissue thinning, which could lead to tissue tearing. This can occur due to postpartum hormonal changes, specifically low estrogen levels. These changes naturally occur for a few months following birth and extend even longer for people who are breastfeeding or chestfeeding or pumping. Additional factors that contribute to pain during sex may include pelvic organ prolapse, the formation of scar tissue and resultant tissue sensitivity and stiffness, menopause, and pelvic muscle tension.

Pain during interceptive sex is common and may be caused by a number of factors, including heightened nervous system sensitivity or elevated tension in the pelvic muscles. Sometimes tension is chronic and habitual and may exist without our awareness. It can develop following an injury, as a result of certain postural habits or misalignment, from repetitive movements or exercise, or from stress. Tension can result from emotional or social factors or from trauma, both physical and psychological. Sometimes, if a painful experience is felt during sex, this can lead to fear and a physiological and emotional feedback loop that creates more tension. You may need to do some more investigating on your own or with the help of a professional to further understand the root cause and address that cause while simultaneously working on lessening the tension.

If you are experiencing pain or are unable to return to having sex, first take a step back and allow time for your body to heal and your hormones to regulate, and to assess your overall well-being. Try not to put pressure on yourself but rather explore ways to be intimate with your partner that don't involve interceptive sex by exploring relaxation techniques like breathing or gentle touch. Smooth, steady breathing plays an immeasurable role in addressing painful intercourse, and practicing this regularly is an important foundational tool. Masturbation may be a safe way to reintroduce touch or intimacy, and keeping the lines of communication open by having regular conversations or seeking out the support and guidance of a sex therapist can be helpful. Graduated dilators can be used to stretch tight tissues over time and can improve your nervous system's response to activity and touch in and around the pelvic area.

When you feel ready to try penetrative intercourse, use plenty of lubrication. A water-soluble lubricant or a natural oil like coconut oil can be used to reduce friction. Note that if you are relying on condoms as your primary form of birth control, all types of oil should be avoided, as this can break down and tear a condom, making it ineffective. Position changes and the use of a support like pillows under your knees or outer hips may feel more supportive and help you relax tense muscles and ease the tendency to grip or guard. Go slowly and back away from anything that feels painful. Many people report that at first they feel pain, but then if they push through, the pain lessens. This can add to a physiological feedback loop, however, that equates any activity in the pelvic region with pain and can add to fear, gripping, and further tension. Again, steady breathing, establishing an open line of communication with your partner, and being willing to go slow or back off will help bring ease to both your body and your mind.

Sex is an intimate act, and for some a highly emotional experience, especially if pain or fear of pain is occurring. Some students have found relief by having a partner help them with their breathing and relaxation, which can be done in any neutral, comfortable position, or even in some of the poses described next, or in the Week 1 sequence such as pose 6, Adho Mukha Vīrāsana, or pose 2, Supta Baddha Koṇāsana. Have your partner place a finger or two on the pelvic floor muscles with very light pressure, and breathe with you, relaxing on the inhalation. This may help reduce some of the painful sensitivity you are feeling as well as allow you and your partner a way to be in an intimate and healing connection together. If you notice you are gripping, holding your breath, or that tension is increasing, then you should back off, as any kind of stress will only reinforce the feedback loop of fear, pain, and tension. Over time, you may be able to soften tension and balance protective responses driven by your nervous system enough that the ability to feel pleasure and ease during sex is restored.

Staying hydrated and doing pelvic floor contractions, if deemed appropriate, can also help with ease of tissue mobility and production of blood flow to the tissues. Additionally, some people benefit from the use of topical estrogen creams prescribed by a provider, which can help reduce hormonal changes like dryness and tissue thinning contributing to friction and pain. If no changes occur and pain with intercourse persists after a few months or multiple attempts, schedule an appointment with your medical provider or a pelvic physical therapist for further assessment and treatment.

## Approach to Āsana

As discussed, there may be many reasons that someone is experiencing pain during intercourse. The reasons may be multifaceted and may include physical, physiological, and psychoemotional factors. Without knowing the individual student, it is hard to give a general set of guidelines. However, pain during interceptive intercourse is a fairly common occurrence, and something that regularly comes up in our courses. In our experience, most often, students who are experiencing pain during interceptive intercourse are also experiencing elevated tension in the pelvic floor muscles, and addressing this tension is vital.

The focus for anyone addressing pelvic floor tension should be on the Week 1 āsanas and the breathwork presented there. Practice each pose with your pelvic floor in mind, and notice whether there are one or two particular poses that help relieve tension. Many students find great relief in Adho Mukha Vīrāsana, as this widens the buttock bones and entire pelvic floor region, and the inhalation can be felt more clearly in the pelvic floor. Prasārita Pādottānāsana, presented in Week 7, pose 7, can also help spread and relieve tension in the pelvic floor. Supta Baddha Koṇāsana is effective because the groins, lower abdomen, and diaphragm are gently stretched, which may allow you to breathe better while also relaxing the pelvic floor. You can also focus on poses that bring you overall relaxation, as this will help you release tension in your overall system.

Additionally, in chapter 1 we give instructions for doing a pelvic self-assessment. If there is pain during penetration, you may have too much pain or be frightened to do a self-assessment. One approach could be to place a finger or two just at the opening of the vagina, or slightly posteriorly at the perineum, and practice breathing here, focusing on relaxation during the inhalation. At first it may feel hard to relax, but with some practice you may start to feel more movement happening in the muscles. Sometimes students report that they can feel some relaxation happening, but then on the exhalation everything grips up again. Practice slowing down the exhalation and slightly resisting the urge to grip. Here, visualizing the pelvic floor releasing, spreading, softening, and so on can be very helpful. Once you feel comfortable with this, you can proceed slowly over several weeks with the rest of the self-assessment. Your approach should be meditative, maintaining a soft approach and rhythmic breath. You can then return to some of the Week 1 poses and practice breathing with a slight amount of pressure from your fingertips on the pelvic floor to notice how the pelvic floor muscles are responding.

# Postpartum Depression and Anxiety

Childbirth is a difficult and exhausting process. Caring for a newborn baby and meeting their needs is challenging and leaves little time for much else. After the birth of a baby, many people experience "baby blues" or feelings of sadness or fatigue. Naturally occurring hormonal changes, and sleep disruption, which is the most common complaint among new parents, can affect your overall health and lead to other symptoms.[26] Typically, baby blues resolve within a few weeks or months and don't interfere with your ability to care for your baby.

Postpartum depression differs from baby blues in that it lasts longer and more severely affects a person's ability to return to normal function. It is characterized by intense feelings of sadness or worthlessness that can make caring for or bonding with your baby difficult. During pregnancy and following birth, tremendous changes are known to occur hormonally, physically, emotionally, and mentally.[27] Additionally, enormous changes occur in a person's familial and interpersonal world. Postpartum depression can affect anyone and typically develops within the first few months following birth, affecting one in seven women. Some risk factors for developing postpartum depression include people who have a history of depression or who have experienced depression and anxiety during pregnancy, lack of sleep, limited physical activity and exercise, lack of social support, high-risk pregnancies that include emergency cesarean delivery, or preterm or low-birth-weight infants.[28]

Understanding signs and symptoms of postpartum depression and anxiety is key in getting the appropriate help. Recognize that symptoms vary and there is a wide range of experiences that postpartum people may be having, regardless of diagnosis. Even recognizing and honoring the changes that you have undergone that may be affecting your emotions, mood, energy, and thoughts can be a good first step in getting the support you need, regardless of whether or not you believe you have postpartum depression. Even if you feel like your symptoms are mild, consider seeking mental health counseling, reaching out to postpartum support groups, talking to your doctor, and talking to trusted friends and family. Talking about your concerns can help you feel like you are not alone in your experience and can help you feel cared for with support. If you are currently pregnant or considering getting pregnant, consider attending childbirth education classes that teach new parents to seek help and support that they might need for childbirth.

## Approach to Āsana

While addressing postpartum depression and anxiety as a whole is outside the scope of this text, we want to include some information about it as it is a common experience that we hear about from students, and we feel that yoga can be a complementary practice that helps the new parent cope with the stresses of caring for a new baby while supporting your physical and mental recovery. The practice of āsana can help balance your hormonal system, bringing your body and mind into better equilibrium. Additionally, lack of sleep can cause and exacerbate postpartum depression and anxiety, and the practice of āsana and prāṇāyāma are useful tools to help relieve fatigue, nourish the nervous system, and aid in better sleep (when you can get it). The suggestions given here are meant to help guide you in caring for yourself, while we also encourage getting help from your primary doctor or ob-gyn, mental health provider, friends and family, and anyone else who can be part of your trusted support network. Remember, it truly takes a village!

One of the most common issues we see is that new parents feel overwhelmed, emotional, and exhausted. The toll that birthing and caring for a new baby takes on the physical, physiological, mental, and emotional body is extreme. Oftentimes, we hear that students feel too tired or too overwhelmed even to begin a practice of yoga. If this sounds like you, we encourage taking a very simple approach! Starting with the Week 1 poses, choose just one pose that you enjoy and can do without too much thought. It can be helpful to leave your mat out with the props already set up so that you can easily get into the pose, especially if you only have five or ten minutes available. Try to do the pose every day, or even multiple times a day, as a way of being in your body, checking in with yourself, and resetting your nervous system. You may be surprised at how helpful even just two or three minutes of practice can be. You may choose to practice like this for some weeks, then gradually add in more poses, but be mindful about not being too hard on yourself or expecting too much. Remember, the pose should be healing and soothing for you, not something more to accomplish when you already have too much to do.

Of the supported, restorative āsanas, the supine chest-openers can be helpful, as they bring spaciousness to the chest and can help you feel uplifted. Supta Baddha Koṇāsana (fig. 2.2) and Setubandha Sarvāṅgāsana (fig. 2.17) both open the chest and soften the diaphragm, aiding in breathing. They help relieve fatigue and bring balance to the endocrine system. Supported forward bends are soothing to the mind and nervous system and may be more appropriate if you are experiencing anxiety. Some experimentation is needed to see which poses actually bring mental relief to you as each person's situation may be different. See Weeks 1 to 3 for more on these āsanas.

Prāṇāyāma can also be helpful for bringing mental relief, quieting the nervous system, and reducing fatigue. Start with a simple Śavāsana, supported on a bolster, along with Ujjāyī stage 1 (even breathing). Gradually add Ujjāyī stage 2 and Bhrāmarī. These are described in Week 3, poses 6, 7, and 8. Ujjāyī stages 3 and 4 can be deeply revitalizing (see B. K. S. Iyengar's *Light on Prāṇāyāma* for instructions). As soon as you are no longer bleeding (about four to six weeks), or longer if you have given birth via cesarean (eight to ten weeks), you can begin your practice of inversions, which are a huge help for the hormonal system and clarifying for the mental body. Śīrṣāsana, Sarvāṅgāsana, and Hālāsana can bring stability and quietness to the mind. Viparīta Karaṇī, supported with a bolster at the wall, and Sarvāṅgāsana supported on a chair are both deeply soothing and are good alternatives if you are feeling particularly fatigued. These inversions are described throughout the text, especially in Weeks 2, 5, and 7. When you are ready, Week 7 begins the practice of Dwipāda Viparīta Daṇḍāsana, supported on a chair, which deepens the effects of the supine chest-opening poses.

# Conclusion

We hope that the information and practices we have presented in this book have been illuminating and helpful. As you continue through your process of healing, you may find specific āsanas, practices, or anatomy begin to take on different meanings, and referring back to information in this book will be useful and clarifying as you continue to experience changes in your body. We encourage you to continue your yoga practice under the guidance of a Certified Iyengar Yoga Teacher. We also encourage you to work with a pelvic floor specialist, and we have included resources for finding these practitioners in your area. Additionally, we have provided further resources for study and learning. We also hope that you will share this information, and help others feel empowered to learn about and communicate about their own pelvic floor experiences. Our hope is that this will encourage people to explore other areas of their health and well-being, as the connections are endless. It can be powerful to become more in touch with your pelvis, and this knowledge may give you a new perspective or insight into other aspects of yourself. Returning to the image of the layers of the onion, the kośas, we hope these new insights ripple out through the many layers of your being.

# APPENDIX: ADDITIONAL RESOURCES

## Books

Natalie Angier, *Woman: An Intimate Geography* (Boston: Mariner Books/ Houghton Mifflin Harcourt, 2014).

Katy Bowman and Christiane Northrup, *Diastasis Recti: The Whole-Body Solution to Abdominal Weakness and Separation* (Chichester, UK: Lotus, 2016).

Blandine Calais-Germain and Allan Kaplan, *The Female Pelvis: Anatomy & Exercises* (Seattle: Eastland, 2003).

Eric Franklin, *Pelvic Power: Mind/Body Exercises for Strength, Flexibility, Posture and Balance for Men and Women* (Hightstown, NJ: Elysian Editions, 2003).

Leslie Howard, *Pelvic Liberation: Using Yoga, Self-Inquiry, and Breath Awareness for Pelvic Health* (Oakland, CA: Leslie Howard Yoga, 2017).

Geeta S. Iyengar, *Yoga: A Gem for Women* (New Delhi: Allied Publishers, 2018).

Geeta S. Iyengar, Rita Keller, and Kerstin Khattab, *Iyengar Yoga for Motherhood: Safe Practice for Expectant & New Mothers* (New York: Sterling, 2010).

Tami Lynn Kent, *Mothering from Your Center: Tapping Your Body's Natural Energy for Pregnancy, Birth, and Parenting* (New York: Atria Paperback, 2013).

Tami Lynn Kent, *Wild Feminine: Finding Power, Spirit & Joy in the Female Body* (London: Simon & Schuster, 2011).

Liz Koch, *The Psoas Book* (Felton, CA: Guinea Pig, 2012).

Amy Stein, *Heal Pelvic Pain* (New York: McGraw-Hill, 2008).

Lois Steinberg and Geeta S. Iyengar, *Geeta S. Iyengar's Guide to a Woman's Yoga Practice* (Urbana, IL: Parvati, 2006).

Kathe Wallace, *Reviving Your Sex Life after Childbirth: Your Guide to Pain-Free and Pleasurable Sex after the Baby* (Seattle: Kathe Wallace, 2014).

# Websites and Blogs

Iyengar Yoga Center of Vermont courses and supplemental materials

 www.iycvt.com/prenatal-postpartum

Find a Certified Iyengar Yoga Teacher

 www.iynaus.org

Find a pelvic floor physical therapist

 www.apta.org

 www.hermanwallace.com

 www.pelvicguru.com

Katy Bowman

 www.nutritiousmovement.com/blog/

Susan Clinton

 www.ltiphysio.com/blog

Ginger Garner

 https://integrativelifestylemed.com/blog

Intimate Rose (pelvic wand, weights)

 www.intimaterose.com

Pelvic Guru

 www.pelvicguru.com

Pelvic Health and Rehab Center

 www.pelvicpainrehab.com

Postpartum Support International

 www.postpartum.net

Lynn Schulte, Institute for Birth Healing

 www.instituteforbirthhealing.com

Lois Steinberg and other books and videos

 www.loissteinberg.com

Julie Wiebe

 www.juliewiebept.com/blog

# Notes

1  Christine Berge, "Heterochronic Processes in Human Evolution: An Onto-genetic Analysis of the Hominid Pelvis," *American Journal of Biological Anthropology* 105:4 (1998), 441–59, https://doi.org/10.1002/(SICI) 1096-8644(199804)105:4<441::AID-AJPA4>3.0.CO;2-R.

2  Jacky Ganguly, Dinkar Kulshreshtha, Mohammed Almotiri, and Mandar Jog, "Muscle Tone Physiology and Abnormalities," *Toxins* 13:4 (2021), 282, https://doi.org/10.3390/toxins13040282.

3  Lorenzo Crumble, "Muscles of the Pelvic Floor," KenHub, August 15, 2023, www.kenhub.com/en/library/anatomy/muscles-of-the-pelvic-floor.

4  Crumble, "Muscles of the Pelvic Floor."

5  Helen E. O'Connell, Kalavampara V. Sanjeevan, and John M. Hutson, "Anatomy of the Clitoris," *Journal of Urology* 174:4 (2005), 1189–95, https://doi.org/10.1097/01.ju.0000173639.38898.cd; Rachel N. Pauls, "Anatomy of the Clitoris and the Female Sexual Response," *Clinical Anatomy* 28:3 (2015), 376–84, https://doi.org/10.1002/ca.22524.

6  Anne Koedt, *The Myth of the Vaginal Orgasm* (Somerville, MA: New England Free Press, 1970); O'Connell et al., "Anatomy of the Clitoris."

7  Marco A. Siccardi and Cristina Valle, *Anatomy, Bony Pelvis and Lower Limb: Pelvic Fascia* (Treasure Island, FL: StatPearls, 2023), www.ncbi.nlm .nih.gov/books/NBK518984.

8  Devyani Hunt, John Clohisy, and Heidi Prather, "Acetabular Labral Tears of the Hip in Women," *Physical Medicine and Rehabilitation Clinics* 18:3 (2007), 497–520, https://doi.org/10.1016/j.pmr.2007.05.007.

9  Laura Jawad, "Pelvic Floor Strength and Function (from Head-to-Toe): Part 2," blog post, LauraJawad.com, March 4, 2019, www.laurajawad.com/post /pelvic-floor-strength-and-function-from-head-to-toe-part-2.

10 Ali Kiapour, Amin Joukar, Hossein Elgafy, Deniz U. Erbulut, Anand K. Agarwal, and Vijay K. Goel, "Biomechanics of the Sacroiliac Joint: Anatomy, Function, Biomechanics, Sexual Dimorphism, and Causes of Pain," *International Journal of Spine Surgery* 14: Suppl. 1 (2020), 3–13, https://doi.org/10.14444/6077.

11 Lynn Schulte, "Open Birthing Pattern Signs and Symptom." Institute for Birth Healing, blog post, n.d., https://instituteforbirthhealing.com/open-birthing-pattern-signs-symptoms.

12 Shahab Shahid, "Rectus Abdominis Muscle," KenHub, July 26, 2023, www.kenhub.com/en/library/anatomy/rectus-abdominis-muscle.

13 Nigel Palastanga and Roger W. Soames, *Anatomy and Human Movement: Structure and Function,* 6th ed. (Edinburgh, UK: Churchill Livingstone, 2012).

14 Gordana Sendić, "Transversus Abdominis Muscle," KenHub, December 5, 2022, www.kenhub.com/en/library/anatomy/transversus-abdominis-muscle.

15 Sean Parker Institute for the Voice, "Normal Voice Function," Weill Cornell Medicine, July 13, 2016, https://voice.weill.cornell.edu/voice-evaluation/normal-voice-function.

16 Niamh Gorman, "Diaphragm," KenHub, June 15, 2023, www.kenhub.com/en/library/anatomy/diaphragm.

17 Teruhisa Komori, "The Relaxation Effect of Prolonged Expiratory Breathing," *Mental Illness* 10:1 (2018), 7669, https://doi.org/10.4081/mi.2018.7669.

18 Matthew D. Barber and Christopher Maher, "Epidemiology and Outcome Assessment of Pelvic Organ Prolapse," *International Urogynecology Journal* 24:11 (2013), 1783–90, https://doi.org/10.1007/s00192-013-2169-9.

19 Julie Wiebe, "What Is a Normal Diastasis?" blog post, *Julie Wiebe PT,* September 3, 2018, www.juliewiebept.com/what-is-a-normal-diastasis.

20 M. Cavalli, A. Aiolfi, P. G. Bruni, L. Manfredini, F. Lombardo, M. T. Bonfanti, D. Bona, and G. Campanelli, "Prevalence and Risk Factors for Diastasis Recti Abdominis: A Review and Proposal of a New Anatomical Variation," *Hernia* 25 (2021), 883–90, https://doi.org/10.1007/s10029-021-02468-8.

21 Gertrude M. Beer, Antonius Schuster, Burkhardt Seifert, Mirjana Manestar, Daniela Mihic-Probst, and Sina A. Weber, "The Normal Width of the

Linea Alba in Nulliparous Women," *Clinical Anatomy* 22:6 (2009), 706–11, https://doi.org/10.1002/ca.20836.

22  Wiebe, "What Is a Normal Diastasis?"

23  Miranda Harvey, "Physical Therapy Guide to Urinary Incontinence," ChoosePT, February 1, 2022, www.choosept.com/guide/physical-therapy -guide-incontinence.

24  Christian Cobreros, "Urinary Frequency," ICS Committees Terminology Discussions, 2018, www.ics.org/committees/standardisation/terminology discussions/urinaryfrequency.

25  American College of Obstetricians and Gynecologists, "When Sex Is Painful," ACOG.org, 2022, www.acog.org/womens-health/faqs/when-sex-is -painful.

26  Sohrab Iranpour, Gholam Reza Kheirabadi, Ahmad Esmaillzadeh, Motahar Heidari-Beni, and Mohammad Reza Maracy, "Association between Sleep Quality and Postpartum Depression," *Journal of Research in Medical Sciences* 21:1 (2016), 110, https://doi.org/10.4103/1735-1995.193500.

27  Saba Mughal, Yusra Azhar, and Waquar Siddiqui, *Postpartum Depression* (Treasure Island, FL: StatPearls, 2022), www.ncbi.nlm.nih.gov/books /NBK519070.

28  Mughal et al., *Postpartum Depression*.

# Bibliography

American College of Obstetricians and Gynecologists. "When Sex Is Painful." ACOG.org. 2022. www.acog.org/womens-health/faqs/when-sex-is-painful.

AnatomyZone. "Pelvic Floor Part 1: The Pelvic Diaphragm—3-D Anatomy Tutorial." YouTube, February 2, 2013. Video, 10:26. www.youtube.com/watch?v=P3BBAMWm2Eo.

AnatomyZone. "Pelvic Floor Part 2: Perineal Membrane and Deep Perineal Pouch—3-D Anatomy Tutorial." YouTube, February 10, 2013. Video, 7:17. www.youtube.com/watch?v=q0Ax3rLFc6M.

Angier, Natalie. *Woman: An Intimate Geography*. Boston: Mariner Books/Houghton Mifflin Harcourt, 2014.

Barber, Matthew D., and Christopher Maher. "Epidemiology and Outcome Assessment of Pelvic Organ Prolapse." *International Urogynecology Journal* 24:11 (2013), 1783–90. https://doi.org/10.1007/s00192-013-2169-9.

Beer, Gertrude M., Antonius Schuster, Burkhardt Seifert, Mirjana Manestar, Daniela Mihic-Probst, and Sina A. Weber. "The Normal Width of the Linea Alba in Nulliparous Women." *Clinical Anatomy* 22:6 (2009), 706–11. https://doi.org/10.1002/ca.20836.

Berge, Christine. "Heterochronic Processes in Human Evolution: An Ontogenetic Analysis of the Hominid Pelvis." *American Journal of Biological Anthropology* 105:4 (1998), 441–59. https://doi.org/10.1002/(SICI)1096-8644(199804)105:4<441::AID-AJPA4>3.0.CO;2-R.

Bowman, Katy, and Christiane Northrup. *Diastasis Recti: The Whole-Body Solution to Abdominal Weakness and Separation*. Chichester, UK: Lotus, 2016.

Brooks, Adam G., and Benjamin G. Domb. "Acetabular Labral Tear and Postpartum Hip Pain." *Obstetrics & Gynecology* 120:5 (2012), 1093–98. https://doi.org/10.1097/aog.0b013e31826fbcc8.

Calais-Germain, Blandine, and Allan Kaplan. *The Female Pelvis: Anatomy & Exercises*. Seattle: Eastland, 2003.

Cavalli, M., A. Aiolfi, P. G. Bruni, L. Manfredini, F. Lombardo, M. T. Bonfanti, D. Bona, and G. Campanelli. "Prevalence and Risk Factors for Diastasis

Recti Abdominis: A Review and Proposal of a New Anatomical Variation." *Hernia* 25 (2021), 883–90. https://doi.org/10.1007/s10029-021-02468-8.

Cobreros, Christian. "Urinary Frequency." ICS Committees Terminology Discussions. 2018. www.ics.org/committees/standardisation/terminology discussions/urinaryfrequency.

Crumble, Lorenzo. "Muscles of the Pelvic Floor." KenHub. August 15, 2023. www.kenhub.com/en/library/anatomy/muscles-of-the-pelvic-floor.

Franklin, Eric. *Pelvic Power: Mind/Body Exercises for Strength, Flexibility, Posture and Balance for Men and Women*. Hightstown, NJ: Elysian Editions, 2003.

Ganguly, Jacky, Dinkar Kulshreshtha, Mohammed Almotiri, and Mandar Jog. "Muscle Tone Physiology and Abnormalities." *Toxins* 13:4 (2021), 282. https://doi.org/10.3390/toxins13040282.

Gorman, Niahm. "Diaphragm." KenHub. June 15, 2023. www.kenhub.com/en /library/anatomy/diaphragm.

Harvey, Miranda. "Physical Therapy Guide to Urinary Incontinence." ChoosePT. February 1, 2022. www.choosept.com/guide/physical-therapy -guide-incontinence.

Howard, Leslie. *Pelvic Liberation: Using Yoga, Self-Inquiry, and Breath Awareness for Pelvic Health*. Oakland, CA: Leslie Howard Yoga, 2017.

Hunt, Devyani, John Clohisy, and Heidi Prather. "Acetabular Labral Tears of the Hip in Women." *Physical Medicine and Rehabilitation Clinics* 18:3 (2007), 497–520. https://doi.org/10.1016/j.pmr.2007.05.007.

Iranpour, Sohrab, Gholam Reza Kheirabadi, Ahmad Esmaillzadeh, Motahar Heidari-Beni, and Mohammad Reza Maracy. "Association between Sleep Quality and Postpartum Depression." *Journal of Research in Medical Sciences* 21:1 (2016), 110. https://doi.org/10.4103/1735-1995.193500.

Iyengar, B. K. S. *Light on Prāṇāyāma: The Yogic Art of Breathing*. Chestnut Ridge, NY: Crossroad, 1981.

Iyengar, Geeta S. *Yoga: A Gem for Women*. New Delhi: Allied Publishers, 2018.

Iyengar, Geeta S., Rita Keller, and Kerstin Khattab. *Iyengar Yoga for Motherhood: Safe Practice for Expectant & New Mothers*. New York: Sterling, 2010.

Jawad, Laura. "Pelvic Floor Strength and Function (from Head-to-Toe): Part 2." Blog post. LauraJawad.com. March 4, 2019. www.laurajawad.com/post /pelvic-floor-strength-and-function-from-head-to-toe-part-2.

Kent, Tami Lynn. *Mothering from Your Center: Tapping Your Body's Natural Energy for Pregnancy, Birth, and Parenting*. New York: Atria Paperback, 2013.

Kent, Tami Lynn. *Wild Feminine: Finding Power, Spirit & Joy in the Female Body*. London: Simon & Schuster, 2011.

Kiapour, Ali, Amin Joukar, Hossein Elgafy, Deniz U. Erbulut, Anand K. Agarwal, and Vijay K. Goel. "Biomechanics of the Sacroiliac Joint: Anatomy, Function, Biomechanics, Sexual Dimorphism, and Causes of Pain." *International Journal of Spine Surgery* 14: Suppl. 1 (2020), 3–13. https://doi.org/10.14444/6077.

Koch, Liz. *The Psoas Book*. Felton, CA: Guinea Pig, 2012.

Koedt, Anne. *The Myth of the Vaginal Orgasm*. Somerville, MA: New England Free Press, 1970.

Komori, Teruhisa. "The Relaxation Effect of Prolonged Expiratory Breathing." *Mental Illness* 10:1 (2018), 7669. https://doi.org/10.4081/mi.2018.7669.

McCarthy, Timothy Patrick, and John McMillian. *The Radical Reader: A Documentary History of the American Radical Tradition*. New York: New Press, 1970. https://archive.org/details/radicalreaderdoc0000unse.

Meijlink, Jane. "Urgency." ICS Committees Terminology Discussions. 2018. www.ics.org/committees/standardisation/terminologydiscussions/urgency.

Mughal, Saba, Yusra Azhar, and Waquar Siddiqui. *Postpartum Depression*. Treasure Island, FL: StatPearls, 2022. www.ncbi.nlm.nih.gov/books/NBK519070.

O'Connell, Helen E., Kalavampara V. Sanjeevan, and John M. Hutson. "Anatomy of the Clitoris." *Journal of Urology* 174:4 (2005), 1189–95. https://doi.org/10.1097/01.ju.0000173639.38898.cd.

O'Sullivan, Susan B., Thomas J. Schmitz, and George D. Fulk. *Physical Rehabilitation*. Philadelphia: F. A. Davis, 2019.

Palastanga, Nigel, and Roger W. Soames. *Anatomy and Human Movement: Structure and Function*, 6th ed. Edinburgh, UK: Churchill Livingstone, 2012.

Pauls, Rachel N. "Anatomy of the Clitoris and the Female Sexual Response." *Clinical Anatomy* 28:3 (2015), 376–84. https://doi.org/10.1002/ca.22524.

Schulte, Lynn. "Open Birthing Pattern Signs and Symptoms." Institute for Birth Healing. Blog post, n.d. https://instituteforbirthhealing.com/open-birthing-pattern-signs-symptoms.

Sean Parker Institute for the Voice. "Normal Voice Function." Weill Cornell Medicine. July 13, 2016. https://voice.weill.cornell.edu/voice-evaluation/normal-voice-function.

Sendić, Gordana. "Transversus Abdominis Muscle." KenHub. December 5, 2022. www.kenhub.com/en/library/anatomy/transversus-abdominis-muscle.

Shahid, Shahab. "Rectus Abdominis Muscle." KenHub. July 26, 2023. www.ken hub.com/en/library/anatomy/rectus-abdominis-muscle.

Siccardi, Marco A., and Cristina Valle. *Anatomy, Bony Pelvis and Lower Limb: Pelvic Fascia*. Treasure Island, FL: StatPearls, 2023. www.ncbi.nlm.nih.gov /books/NBK518984.

Stein, Amy. *Heal Pelvic Pain*. New York: McGraw-Hill, 2008.

Steinberg, Lois, and Geeta S. Iyengar. *Geeta S. Iyengar's Guide to a Woman's Yoga Practice*. Urbana, IL: Parvati Productions, 2006.

Wallace, Kathe. *Reviving Your Sex Life after Childbirth: Your Guide to Pain-Free and Pleasurable Sex after the Baby*. Seattle: Kathe Wallace, 2014.

Wiebe, Julie. "What Is a Normal Diastasis?" blog post, *Julie Wiebe PT*. September 3, 2018. www.juliewiebept.com/what-is-a-normal-diastasis.

# Index

energy
downward-moving, 194
and mūla bandha, 88
upward-moving, 94, 109
and vāyus, 122
estrogen, low, 209
exertion, 198–199
exhalation
during exertions, 198–199
long, 97
and pelvic floor contraction, 70, 86–87
Expansion of the Life Force, 97
Extended Triangle Pose, 108–109, 126, 127
external oblique muscles, 41, 42

**F**

face, softening the, 65
fascia
of the hip joint, 33
linea alba, 196, 198, 199
perineal membrane, 16
restoring tension to, 198, 199
whole bodily, 13
fatigue, relieving, 97, 213, 214
femur, 30, 31, 34
fight-flight-freeze response, 46, 48
flatulence, vaginal, 207–208
forward bends
Adho Mukha Swastikāsana, 61
Adho Mukha Vīrāsana, 62
for depression/anxiety, 213–214
Jānu Śirṣāsana, 90, 94
muscles involved in, 41, 42
Paśchimottānāsana, 113–115
frontal plane, 8

**G**

gender inclusivity, 2, 7
genitals, 15
glans clitoris, 29
gluteal muscles, 36–38, 73, 76, 137, 144, 175
gluteus maximus, 36, 37
gluteus medius, 36, 37
gluteus minimus, 36
Gomukhāsana Arms (Cow-Faced Pose), 105–106
greater trochanter, 31
The Great Seal, 91–94

**H**

Half Bridge Pose, 143–146
Half Headstand, 132–134

Half Intense Stretch, 72–73
Half Moon Pose, 111–112, 127
Half Plow Pose, 78–79
hamstrings, 38, 130, 137
Head-to-Knee Pose, 90–91
healing
of the clitoris, 29–30
common postpartum symptoms, 181
of organ prolapse, 193
patience with, 101, 209
of the pelvic floor, 2–3
personalized timing for, 51–52
and rest, 54
and scar tissue, 184
from surgery, 188, 190
three phases of pelvic, 3, 4
through the kośas, 4–5
heart openers, 169, 170
hernia, 127, 143, 201–203
hesitancy, urinary, 205
hip compaction, 74
hip joint
anatomy of, 30–38
assessment of, 8
compacting, 108, 109, 130, 157
imbalance in, 101
stabilizing of, 156
*See also* iliopsoas
hormones
balancing, 169, 170, 174, 213
inversions for, 214
and ligamentous laxity, 33, 192, 207
and linea alba elasticity, 197
and postpartum depression, 212
and vaginal changes, 209
hysterectomy, 207

**I**

iliacus, 141
iliopsoas, 43, 44, 45, 46, 141, 146
ilium, 8
imbalance
alignment to correct, 69
in bridge pose, 145
compensation for muscular, 101
correcting hip, 111
shoulder, 107
incontinence, 1, 203–204
individualization, 4
inhalation, 69–70
inlet, pelvic, 12
insomnia, 97
instability, 11, 78, 190

# About the Authors

**Rebecca Weisman** is a Certified Iyengar Yoga Teacher and the director of the Iyengar Yoga Center of Vermont. She has been a devoted student of Iyengar Yoga for over twenty years and has a passion for all eight limbs of the yoga system as well as a deep love of experiential anatomy and therapeutic yoga. She is devoted to her main teacher, Patricia Walden, and has studied extensively with other senior Iyengar teachers as well as directly with the Iyengar family in Pune, India. Having discovered yoga at a young age, Rebecca initially was drawn to its healing elements as she recovered from serious physical ailments, finding the precision and depth of the Iyengar method to be uniquely beneficial. Rebecca was also initially drawn to the philosophy of yoga and the mental effects of the practice, and used yoga as a way out of mental and emotional turmoil.

She is guided in her teaching with the belief that the therapeutic benefits of the āsana, prāṇāyāma, and philosophy of yoga can be felt even for a beginner student, and her teaching is infused with a love of both the science and art of yoga. She teaches prenatal and postpartum yoga and works with individuals with diverse issues, including fatigue, depression, chronic illness, chronic pain, lower back pain and sciatica, hip, knee, shoulder, and neck problems, injury recovery, anxiety, and blood pressure and immune system disorders. She is also a mother of two young children and brings to her work her experience of the physical aspects of pregnancy, childbirth, and postpartum recovery as well as the humor, patience, and ease needed to parent. In addition to practice and teaching, Rebecca has a background in art and maintains a vibrant art practice, which includes many of the illustrations for *Yoga for Pelvic Floor and Postpartum Health*.

**Meagen Satinsky** earned a master's degree in physical therapy from Simmons College in 2000. She has worked as a PT in various health care settings around the country, from inpatient rehab at MossRehab in Philadelphia to outpatient treatment at Evolution PT & Yoga in Burlington, Vermont, and everything in between. Following the path to merge the science and art of healing has been an intensive study both professionally and personally. Five years into her PT career, Meagen sustained an injury while working, resulting in nagging and sometimes debilitating lower back pain. As part of her efforts to heal, she took her first yoga class. It left her feeling curious, refreshed, and excited about the roots and depth of study passed down through generations of devoted teachers and students. She naturally made connections and filled in gaps in her own studies using ideas and teachings of both Eastern and Western approaches to the human body.

In 2006 she earned a certification with Corina Benner and Jill Manning through Wake Up Yoga in Philadelphia, and continued to seek ways to blend these practices in meaningful ways. After completing her first PT Pelvic Health course in 2011, she knew right away just how healing and important this work would prove to be in her personal and professional life, for she began to see and understand her own back pain through a different lens. For her, this was the missing link! An experiential learner at heart, Meg traveled to Mysore, India, in 2013 to further her personal study of yoga āsana, philosophy, music, and language. Upon her return to the United States and shortly after landing in Vermont, in 2014 she attended her first ever Iyengar Yoga class with Rebecca Weisman at the Iyengar Yoga Center of Vermont. Many of the teachings within the Iyengar Yoga system, the creative and intelligent use of props as well as breathing and mindfulness practices, were a natural fit and complemented Meg's approach to health and wellness.

In 2014 she earned a certification in Professional Medical Yoga Therapy with Ginger Garner, DPT, and began to integrate this work into her practice at Evolution PT & Yoga with a community of creative and inspiring therapists, teachers, students, clients, and friends. Through her regular practice she has experienced many changes in support of her physical, energetic, emotional, and mental bodies. Today she is the proud owner of Meagen Satinsky PT, PLLC at Pelvic Health in South Burlington, Vermont, where she aims to listen, collaborate, support, and empower all individuals with their individualized pelvic health and orthopedic wellness needs. She feels lucky to share her passion with others.

# About North Atlantic Books

North Atlantic Books (NAB) is an independent, nonprofit publisher committed to a bold exploration of the relationships between mind, body, spirit, and nature. Founded in 1974, NAB aims to nurture a holistic view of the arts, sciences, humanities, and healing. To make a donation or to learn more about our books, authors, events, and newsletter, please visit www.northatlanticbooks.com.